FIT *and* FABULOUS in **15** MINUTES

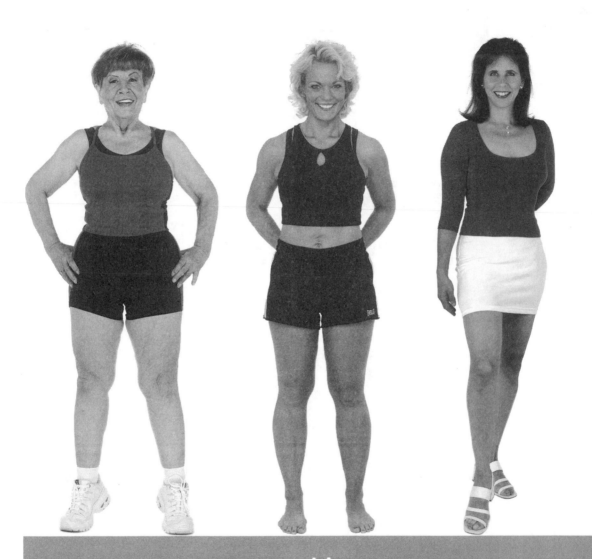

BALLANTINE BOOKS

New York

FIT *and* FABULOUS *in* 15 MINUTES

Teresa Tapp
with Barbara Smalley

Author's Note: *Fit and Fabulous in 15 Minutes* proposes a program of exercise recommendations for the reader to follow. However, you should consult a qualified medical professional (and, if you are pregnant, your obstetrician) before starting this or any other fitness program. As with any diet or exercise program, if at any time you experience any discomfort, stop immediately and consult your physician.

2006 Ballantine Books Trade Paperback Edition

Published in the United States by Ballantine Books,
an imprint of The Random House Publishing Group,
a division of Random House, Inc., New York.

BALLANTINE and colophon are registered trademarks of Random House, Inc.

Originally published in hardcover in the United States by Ballantine Books, an imprint of The Random House Publishing Group, a division of Random House, Inc., in 2006.

ISBN 978-0-345-48404-8

Printed in the United States of America

www.ballantinebooks.com

15 14 13 12 11 10

Book design by Mary A. Wirth

In memory of Corenna Booten Tapp, Minnie Endsley, and Joy Holiday,
whose words of wisdom were instrumental in developing my passion
to live life with purpose and to always look for the positive
in any challenge.

I dedicate this book to God for giving me the ability to speak,
educate, and elevate. He has blessed me in so many ways,
and I am forever grateful for His unconditional love,
support, and guidance in helping me understand
the power of movement within the human body.

Acknowledgments

Writing these acknowledgments is difficult because after 30 years of living, learning, and researching the power of T-Tapp, it is impossible to mention all those who have helped, inspired, and influenced me along the way. However, I would like to recognize those who directly helped bring T-Tapp to print.

I've always known that writing a book about T-Tapp would not be easy, but writing and publishing it within a year would have been impossible had it not been for my co-author, Barbara Smalley, my publicist, Kitty Eatherly, and our incredible agent, Heide Lange. I will never forget how it all began in NYC, the long hours at WaterMark, or the multiple phone calls in between. Kitty, your title as publicist doesn't nearly indicate the amount of work you did in helping to write this book, and no one can type as fast as I can talk except you.

I'd like to thank my editor, Caroline Sutton, who realized and believed in T-Tapp right from the start and saw it through to completion.

Additionally, I want to thank my staff for maintaining business as usual at the T-Tapp office without my presence and for providing excellent service and support for T-Tappers when needed. A special note of appreciation to Lauren Lucernoni and her support team of Casey Ellis,

Jennifer Decker, and Brian Hashey for helping to deliver all the testimonial images in proper format and on time for production.

Thanks to my fellow daybreak divas and dude (Alex, Barb, Berei, Brenda, Cheryl, Jeanne, Jill, Judy, Margie, Rhonda, Scott, and Theresa) for your supportive spirit. Our 6 a.m. workouts allowed me to start each morning with humor and clarity of mind along with energy to stay productive all day. But an extra thank-you to Berei for calling me each morning to make sure I was there!

Many thanks to my T-Tapp Certified Trainers for sharing my passion in helping others build better bodies. Your quality of instruction has helped T-Tapp expand with outstanding clinics and classes across the world.

Above all, thanks to everyone who has spread the news about T-Tapp. Your word-of-mouth advertising has inspired many to join the T-Tapp team and has fueled T-Tapp to grow with strength and stability. I am especially thankful for those who were willing to share their success stories with pictures in this book. Results always speak louder than words, and your before-and-after pictures are sure to motivate many!

I am indebted to Dave Monroe, our photographer, for his extra efforts in bringing each exercise to life. I appreciate you and will never forget those long days of editing at your studio with Buddy and Nala-Linn.

To my parents, sister, brother, nieces, nephews, and all my in-laws— thanks for your encouragement and for understanding my absence from family events while I worked on this project.

But most of all, special thanks to my best friend and partner in life, Mark Dinkel, for your love, support, and patience during my relentless drive with T-Tapp. I love you and thank you for providing me "heaven on earth" and for teaching me the importance of play. I promise, deadlines are over.

And I am grateful to my two precious pets, Ivy and Buddy, for bringing such joy and peace to my life. Nothing compares to horse kisses or puppy play to make me smile at the end of each day.

—*Teresa Tapp*

first met Teresa Tapp when I was assigned to write an article about T-Tapp for *Woman's World* magazine. After several in-depth interviews with her—and hearing many of her success stories—I couldn't believe she had not shared her workout with the rest of the world by writing a book. When she agreed to let me help her with this project, I felt extremely honored, and what began as a business collaboration quickly blossomed into a friendship. Teresa, what a privilege it has been getting to know you. Your knowledge of the human body and your expertise in health and wellness never cease to amaze me!

There are just two names listed on the cover of this book, but in all fairness, Kitty Eatherly's name belongs there as well. Aside from being a crackerjack publicist, Kitty was instrumental not only in helping us to meet tight deadlines, but also in coordinating T-Tapp contests that enabled us to share our latest and greatest success stories. Kitty, it's rare to click so quickly with someone, and I'll always treasure our work sessions at "the land." (Oh no, the laptop crashed again!)

This book never would have been published were it not for our agent, Heide Lange, who literally sold the idea by becoming a T-Tapper herself and wowing her colleagues in the publishing world.

Sincere thanks to our editor, Caroline Sutton, who realized this book's potential from the beginning and edited it with pure professionalism and a (welcome) sense of humor. The Random House team is also impressive. We are fortunate to have such an outstanding group of professionals in our corner and owe a debt of thanks to Christina Duffy and everyone in the production department there as well.

I am especially grateful to my husband, Tim, and sons, Logan and Ben, who have helped me to maintain a sense of balance throughout this project. I am also grateful to my mother, Zelda Steinberg, and my sisters, Avra Hawkins and Dale Steinberg, for providing me with a lifetime of love and support.

How could a book be written without the support of close friends? It can't! So, many thanks to Laurie Fowler, Connie Glaser, Judy and

Dan Hees, Lynn Massey, Kelly Rodgers, Gail and Kim Stearman, and the whole gang at the Prescription Gym for always listening and for providing much-needed distractions.

Finally, a special thank-you to my late father, M. K. Steinberg, who always believed in me and whose kindness to others continues to inspire me.

—Barbara Smalley

Contents

FIT *and* FABULOUS *in* 15 MINUTES

Hi, I'm Teresa Tapp

Fit and fabulous in fifteen minutes? I know what you're thinking. It sounds too good to be true and even a bit sensationalized, doesn't it? Well, get ready, because in this book, you're going to discover that "yes you can!"

Welcome to T-Tapp, the wellness workout that works wonders for your body, mind, and spirit. I take a rehabilitative approach to fitness and spent nine years creating this workout—plus over two decades perfecting it. As you learn the exercises in this book, you'll immediately feel the difference between T-Tapp and other workouts you've tried, and you'll experience head-to-toe results like never before. You'll also discover how less is more, since T-Tapp's special form and techniques maximize muscle development, enabling your body to shed inches in record time. In fact, the stronger you get, the more you get out of T-Tapp—and the less you have to do it to stay in shape!

But first I thought you might want to know a little about me, how I created this workout, and why I'm so excited to be sharing it with you.

I am five feet seven inches tall, weigh about 130 pounds, and wear a size six. I haven't gone to a gym, lifted a single weight, or done any other exercise program except T-Tapp for over twenty years. Even then, I don't work out every day—and you won't have to, either. In fact, T-Tapp workouts are based on *quality,* not quantity, with movements designed to give maximum results in minimum time.

I'm a huge jazz and blues fan and love to dance. But there is no music in T-Tapp, and despite its name, tap dancing is not part of this workout. T-Tapp is aerobic, yet there is no jumping or running involved—which means no stress on your joints. You won't lift a single weight, yet you'll still reap all the benefits of strength training, such as stronger bones and prevention of osteoporosis. That's because T-Tapp's focus is on using your own *body* as the machine.

Moreover, because T-Tapp is *no*-impact, you can perform these exercises for life—no matter your age or physical condition. In fact, there are hundreds of T-Tappers who are well into their seventies, eighties, and nineties!

I love red wine and firmly believe that life is too short to deny yourself good food. Most days I try to eat a balanced diet, but I cheat frequently. I can rarely drive by a Krispy Kreme doughnut shop when the red light is on, which means the doughnuts are hot and fresh—yum! And my office staff must occasionally hide almond M&Ms from me. The good news is that T-Tapp helps to reset your metabolism to burn at a faster rate, so you can eat, cheat, and still lose inches!

I'm an outdoor person. I love riding my horse, Ivy, and playing with my beloved bichon, Buddy. Most weekends you'll find me digging in the dirt, planting flowers, and cutting the grass with a push mower. But I'm just as happy curled up on the couch reading anything about the human body. Hours become minutes when I discover new research and studies that reveal statistical patterns about how the human body works. In my opinion, the body is an amazing machine that can rebuild wellness—and wellness is what I am most passionate about in life.

This passion began, believe it or not, at the tender age of five—

and for tragic reasons. That's when I lost my mother, Corenna, to brain cancer. She was twenty-nine at the time and had endured four operations and two years of grueling radiation and chemotherapy. Because of her illness, I spent much of my early childhood hanging out in hospitals. As I watched my mother suffer, I dreamed of becoming a doctor when I grew up so that I could find a cure for cancer.

But there were silver linings to all this sadness. Experiencing the loss of a loved one at such an early age gave me an insight into wellness that was far beyond my years. And as my mother's condition deteriorated, I instinctively learned to value my own health and recognized the importance of listening to—and taking care of—my own body.

My mother battled cancer with courage and humor, always seeing the glass as half full. When the side effects of chemotherapy forced her to wear a wig, for example, she'd laugh and say, "I may have lost all my hair, but now I get to be a blonde!" Fortunately, I inherited her knack for finding the positive in every negative situation, and her legacy has served me well.

For instance, in high school, a nasty fall from a balance beam in gym class chipped three vertebrae in the mid-lumbar region of my back. That injury, coupled with the scoliosis I'd suffered from since childhood, often left me nearly paralyzed with pain. Yet instead of listening to my doctor, who recommended bed rest, I listened to that inner voice in the back of my head that said I needed to move my body to find relief. After weeks of experimenting with all kinds of muscle movements, I was elated to discover exercises that would alleviate my back pain. I was equally thrilled to discover that I'd shrunk several inches in the process—what a bonus!

At eighteen, I enrolled at Waubonsee Community College, where I received an associate's degree in science before transferring to Eastern Illinois University as a pre-med major. There, while pursuing a bachelor of science degree in exercise physiology (with an emphasis on public health and education), I did extensive volunteer work with cancer patients who were undergoing radiation and chemotherapy. When these women consistently complained of nausea and edema, I was able to further test the effectiveness of my exercises. I had a hunch that certain muscle movements would bring these women relief, and I was right. But the big discovery here was that *sequence* seemed to matter. In other words, performing my exercises in a specific order helped to diminish puffiness and nausea so dramatically that it appeared to be eliminating toxins from the body.

I realized that I was definitely on to something when every single patient who was using my exercises—in the right order—reported significant relief and reduced swelling. This was extremely exciting for these women, because it meant their bodies would be better able to endure treatments to fight this horrible disease. Needless to say, they were also elated about tightening, toning, and losing a few inches along the way.

While working with these patients, I found a suspicious lump— about the size of a walnut—under my right armpit. I was nineteen at the time, and given my family history, my peers and professors (many of whom were physicians) advised, "Have it removed immediately, or you could be dead by age thirty." In those days, surgery was the answer to every bump and lump, for fear these would turn into cancer and metastasize. But I wasn't alarmed. I had noticed that if I didn't get enough sleep, ate too much sugar, or drank one too many glasses of wine, that lump would swell. But when I performed the same sequence of movements I was teaching the cancer patients I was working with, the lump drastically shrank. Oddly enough, this lump had become a barometer for my body, indicating my level of fitness and wellness. So I was worried that if doctors removed it, I would lose my "radar" and have trouble listening to my body.

Of course, I advise everyone to have any lumps thoroughly checked by a health care professional, as I did. Fortunately, in my case, there was no need for surgery. In fact, that lump is still with me today and continues to fluctuate in size, depending on what I've been eating or drinking and how much—or how little—I've been working out.

After I graduated from college, Eastern Illinois University offered me a graduate assistantship to study the specific changes that seem to occur in women's bodies every decade in terms of weight gain. I had always been curious about the "freshman fifteen"—you know, those extra pounds most students tend to pack on in their first year of college. I knew it wasn't just due to pizza and beer, because even coeds who didn't drink or eat a lot of fast food were experiencing weight gain, or what I call the notorious "fat shift."

My study wasn't limited to college students; it also included older pre- and postmenopausal women. This research empowered me to understand the connection between internal muscle development and how we metabolize calories at rest. I quickly realized the effectiveness of T-Tapp moves in helping the body maintain optimal metabolic processing regardless of age, and that made me even more passionate about my program. Another finding that blew me away: 100 percent of these women reported the results of better hormonal balance—far fewer cramps, bloating, hot flashes, and mood swings—after trying my workout.

I had every intention of completing my master's degree and applying to medical school, but tuition money was tight. About that time, the fashion industry made me an offer I couldn't refuse: the chance to work as a new-face developer and booker, preparing new models for the business. One of the side benefits—and, honestly, one of the main reasons I took this job—was being able to work in Germany, where they were years ahead of America in terms of holistic and rehabilitative approaches to health and wellness. During my tenure, I trained thousands of models—even some supermodels—and realized that it doesn't matter what you weigh. Inches count, pounds don't. In fact, no models I worked with were ever put on a scale. Instead, their measurements were their calling cards. And if the clothes didn't fit, a model didn't work.

That's why with T-Tapp, I'm going to tell you to ignore the scale and focus solely on inch loss. I don't want you to obsess too much about tag sizes, either, because no matter how much you work out, your body type and structure may simply not enable you to ever wear a size four or six. Looking your best is more about having everything fit, firm, and in the right place. Trust me, I've seen my share of skinny but lumpy size two models who didn't look nearly as good as a size sixteen T-Tapper who is fit and firm!

I shared my exercises with these models and not only trimmed their trouble spots but boosted their energy levels. They loved my workout, because it delivered inch-loss results *fast*. It was also no-fuss. Requiring a mere four square feet of space, these moves were perfect for models accustomed to living out of hotel rooms. What's more, the same movements I'd been using for years to manage my back pain helped these models alleviate muscle soreness brought on by grueling twelve-hour shoots and the contortionist-like poses that photographers often required them to hold for long periods of time.

Working in the fashion industry was never part of my game plan, but in hindsight, this priceless hands-on experience allowed me to gather valuable statistical data. Working with models of different shapes, sizes, heritages, and figure problems was like taking a course in physiology. Based on what I learned, I was able to fine-tune many of my existing exercises, as well as develop new moves that would trim and tone regardless of one's body type. Working abroad also exposed me to cutting-edge research in the areas of nutrition and botanical supplements.

The models I worked with often called me "Mother T," and to this day, many continue to stay trim and toned using T-Tapp moves. In a recent interview with fashion editor Evelyn Theiss, for example, I learned that many of today's runway models routinely perform one of my energizing signature moves—called Hoe Downs—prior to every fashion show. Many also rely on T-Tapp moves to quickly whip them into shape for swimsuit and lingerie catalog shoots (like Victoria's Secret), as well as the all-important designer fashion shows, where audiences are virtually a who's who of the fashion world.

After a decade of globetrotting, I was ready to return to the States, settle down, and share the benefits of my workout with women and men from all walks of life. I moved to Tampa Bay, Florida, and spent the next five years copyrighting my exercises and reconnecting with the medical community. Various psychologists, oncologists, and doctors of osteopathic medicine referred patients to me for rehabilitative training. These clients faced a variety of challenges—from cancer to eating disorders to manic-depression—and it was incredibly satisfying to see that T-Tapping could make a difference in their lives. During this time, I also worked one-on-one as a personal trainer with a handful of models, celebrities, and everyday women who were anxious to achieve their fitness goals.

T-Tapp has always been about empowering others, so typically I would work with clients for only two weeks, making sure they knew how to T-Tapp on their own before letting them go. Despite this policy, my waiting list for new clients soon swelled to eight months. So much for reaching the masses! Realizing that I was maxed out and could help only so many people in a day, I knew it was time for a new strategy.

That's when *Women's Fitness International* magazine approached me about becoming a contributing editor. I saw this as a golden opportunity both to educate scores of women and men and to showcase my exercise program. With each bimonthly article I wrote, I would share my thoughts and theories on health and nutrition, as well as feature one exercise in depth. Reader response was phenomenal, so I began filming my first at-home fitness video, which the magazine agreed to pitch. It was called *The Super Fat Burning Inch Loss System*. A mouthful, I know, but customers loved the workout.

Two years later, I decided to take advantage of the Internet boom and establish a Web site. I filled it with educational articles and set up a message board to encourage T-Tappers to communicate with one another. I created more fitness videos and offered these for sale at my Web site. I also finally decided to call my workout T-Tapp. Doing so enabled me to brand the name—not to mention that using the Tapp name made my father very proud.

Meanwhile, *Women's Fitness International* was sold, and I realized it was time to branch out on my own. I was eager to contribute articles and exercises to non-fitness magazines anyway, as well as spread the word about T-Tapp through other media.

During sweeps week of 2000, KTRK, the ABC News affiliate in Houston, Texas, ran a "Yes You Can" T-Tapp Challenge, which followed eight women over a two-week period. When every single participant lost a clothing size—without dieting—other ABC affiliates picked up the story. I credit WPIV in Philadelphia with putting T-Tapp on the map. In response to its broadcast, I gained twenty thousand new customers in the first week alone!

Then I spent eighteen months touring small towns from coast to coast, sharing the T-Tapp workout with women and men nationwide through free "Yes You Can" seminars. As you know, wellness is my passion, so I found this experience to be extremely rewarding.

Today, there are hundreds of thousands of women and men around the world who T-Tapp. My workout has earned kudos because:

1. It can be done anywhere—even on the road when you're traveling.
2. You need only four square feet of space to do it.
3. There's no need to join a gym.
4. You don't have to invest in a single piece of equipment— not even a stretchy band or hand weights.

Fair warning: T-Tapp moves may *look* simple, but make no mistake about it—there's a lot more going on than meets the eye. Granted, you'll never do more than eight repetitions of any exercise, but these comprehensive movements always work five to seven muscles at once. Plus you'll be finished with your workout in anywhere from fifteen to forty-five minutes. Nevertheless, T-Tapp is an intense little workout that delivers big results—inside and out. I'm pleased that my straightforward, no-nonsense approach has earned me a reputation for "getting real"—as in *real* results for *real* women (and men) *real* fast. Perhaps that's why some refer to me as the "Dr. Phil of fitness."

Indeed, with T-Tapp, you don't have to wait months to see dramatic changes in the mirror. Whether you're twenty-something or over sixty, fit or out of shape, you will emerge slimmer and trimmer in just two weeks. The *average* T-Tapper reports losses of at least one clothing size in four weeks; many others drop a size in just fourteen days—all without changing their diet.

After T-Tapping for two weeks, you're going to feel terrific, too. I take a rehabilitative approach to fitness, which means that the moves I've created are designed to help your body help itself repair, rebuild, and rejuvenate. In addition to shedding inches, you'll feel like the Energizer bunny. You'll also stand taller, feel stronger, and enjoy greater mental clarity.

More good news: this functional fitness approach not only makes T-Tapp workouts safe for many people with shoulder, hip, knee, neck, and back concerns, but it often frees them from the chronic pain they've been living with. Even those with chronic illnesses—such as fibromyalgia, lupus, chronic fatigue syndrome, and multiple sclerosis—have reported wonderful results with T-Tapp. People dealing with type 2 diabetes, high blood pressure, arthritis, and high cholesterol have also reported great improvement from T-Tapping. But don't take my word for it. Amazing success stories from real T-Tappers who have enjoyed enormous wellness and aesthetic benefits from these exercises are featured throughout this book. I'm certain their "it worked for me" narratives will motivate and inspire you to join their ranks.

I've designed T-Tapp to be a left-brain/right-brain, mind/body workout, so expect your mental clarity to soar. Since each side of the brain controls the other side of the body, using both sides of the brain when you exercise results in the rapid release of neurotransmitters, which not only increases mental alertness but uses more energy and burns more fat.

With T-Tapp, I'm also going to teach you how to rediscover your own inner voice. I believe we all have one; we just get too busy with life and have a tendency to stop listening to our bodies. For total wellness, however, I believe it's important to connect mind and body, and T-Tapp will show you how to do just that—and feel better than ever.

As you read this book, I'll be your personal trainer, coach, cheerleader, and educator every step of the way. In Chapter 2, I'll elaborate on how and why T-Tapp is more comprehensive than other workouts. I'll also make promises and share success stories that may sound too good to be true. Then I'll show you that yes, you can be your *own* success story!

In Chapter 3, you'll learn the primary principles and basic prerequisites of T-Tapping. Before lacing up your cross-trainers and getting started, it's extremely important that you read all of the information presented here. Otherwise, you may not see the speedy results that T-Tapp promises.

Chapter 4 introduces my wellness workout, the Basic Plus Workout. Designed primarily for beginners and to help the fit get fitter, it delivers inch loss as well as improved health and wellness. This quickie workout tightens and tones, strengthens and stretches, de-stresses and energizes—plus saves time. It takes just fifteen minutes to complete, yet still provides cardiac conditioning and improved circulation to leave you with an "I kick butt" glow.

My Total Workout is presented in Chapter 5. These moves, when performed in combination with the moves from the Basic Plus Workout, deliver faster and more dramatic inch loss and will wow you with their fat-melting powers. The Total Workout really concentrates on the core and delivers body sculpting in addition to the benefits of a full session of aerobics, as well as a full session of traditional strength training. From start to finish, it will sculpt your muscles, strengthen your center, and speed up your metabolism so that you'll see results—and fast.

It's important to remember that T-Tapp's focus is not on losing weight but on shedding inches and completely reshaping your body so that you look and feel better. Naturally, as soon as you start losing inches, the pounds typically follow. That's because once your developing muscles get hungry, they will feast on the best fuel of all: *your* body fat.

That said, taking a commonsense approach to eating *will* help you shrink faster and feel better. To help you accomplish that, check out my God-Made, Man-Made Food Plan in Chapter 6, which allows you to splurge and splurge again every three days and still reach your goal. You won't have to count a single calorie or fat gram or endure a single hunger pang. You won't have to eliminate carbs, either, or give up *any* of your favorite foods. Rather, the God-Made, Man-Made Food Plan is a straightforward approach that trains your body to better process man-made foods. By eating only healthy and nutritious—God-made—foods for two days, you help your body rebuild body systems such as assimilation, digestion, and particularly elimination. In fact, once your body gets into the habit of eating better foods, it's easier for it to get rid of any fats and toxins you consume by eating man-made foods on your cheat days. Thus, you keep your weight under control without feeling deprived.

If you still have questions after trying all the exercises in this book and checking out the God-Made, Man-Made Food Plan, flip to Chapter 7 for answers. Here you'll find a collection of the inquiries I hear most. Finally, for further motivation and inspiration, check out Chapter 8, entitled "Encore! Encore!" This collection of T-Tapp success stories features a variety of body types and stages of development, and I'm certain you will find at least one—if not several—success stories you can relate to.

Gregory Heigh, host of the nationally syndicated radio show *Talking Health,* recently described T-Tapp as "the most impressive exercise program I have seen in my thirty-plus years of practice in the field of health and fitness. Never have I seen such a well-designed program that literally reshapes the body as it resets the metabolism to burn at a faster rate. This may very well be the most effective exercise routine on record."

Once you begin T-Tapping, I think you'll agree. No matter what shape you're in now, you'll end up with a leaner, stronger, and more flexible body—and you'll feel the difference inside as well. Remember, I'm an educator at heart, and my goal is to give you all the tools you need to help your body help itself be trim and feel terrific. But, again, please pay careful attention to all the detailed instructions I've provided, because with T-Tapp, proper form is imperative for optimal results.

So, what are you waiting for? You've got to move it to make it happen, and it's never too early or too late to get started. Enjoy—and be *your* best!

Yes You Can!

It's time to stop the old way of thinking about health and fitness. The idea that you have to work out every day for an hour or more—and go to a gym or purchase pricey equipment to do it—is what's keeping a lot of folks on the couch.

You've probably heard the latest statistics: nearly two-thirds of Americans age twenty and up are overweight, and 30 percent are obese, according to the National Center for Health Statistics. These excess pounds and inches have led to a near-epidemic of type 2 diabetes, not to mention the chronic pain that often comes with carrying around too much weight. If you're a baby boomer, menopause is often the culprit behind your extra "baggage." As estrogen decreases, bones lose density and metabolism slows. All too often, the pudge won't budge— even for those who diet and spend hours at the gym.

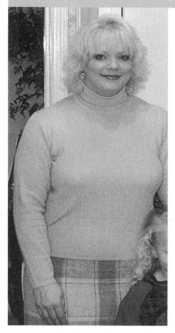

Holli Greene

The New Year's resolution that turned her life around

In January 2003, I went on a field trip with my daughter to the circus. I can remember sitting there thinking about how happy I should be but how miserable I was. My marriage was failing, I had financial problems, and I was very unhappy with myself. Little wonder—at the time, I weighed 215 pounds and wore a size sixteen. That day, I decided to make some New Year's resolutions. I vowed to do whatever it took to improve my home life and finances and to lose weight and keep it off.

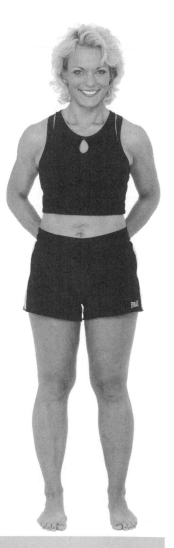

I began T-Tapping soon after that and started with a fourteen-day boot camp. I didn't follow a specific eating plan. Instead, I just tried to cut down on fat and calories and avoid fried foods and desserts. I also drank a gallon of water every day.

By the end of May, I was divorced, had lost sixty pounds, and was wearing a size six. I had never been that small in my entire adult life! Everyone kept asking me how I could eat the foods I did and still maintain my weight. And they couldn't believe that I could maintain my results by working out just one or two times a week.

I have kept the weight off for nearly two years and am now engaged to a wonderful man. I am happier than I have ever been.

T-Tapp has the power to change all that, because it delivers awesome results to everyone—regardless of age, gender, fitness level, or body type. In fact, with T-Tapp, there's really no excuse not to be in the best shape of your life! You only need four square feet of space, and there's no equipment required. You don't need music, and you don't even have to change your diet to see great results. Best of all, T-Tapp is a workout that you will never outgrow. Indeed, the stronger you become, the more control you will have over muscle contractions, so the more you get out of the workout.

Even the very fit can be challenged and see visible results quickly with T-Tapp. In preliminary tests conducted at a prestigious U.S. aerobic institution, even weight trainers and exercise instructors were challenged, easily hitting 75 percent of their target heart rate while doing my forty-five-minute beginner-level workout.

If you're like most people, you've already tried at least five other exercise programs, as well as every new diet fad to hit the market. Great! What that tells me is you're definitely committed to being fit and that you are what I call "exercise educated." That means you understand more about your body than most people do, and you know how the body works. But even if you're a novice, I realize that without immediate results, most people aren't motivated to continue with *any* exercise program. Fortunately, with T-Tapp, that's not a problem.

What sets T-Tapp apart from other exercise programs is how quickly it works and how terrific it makes you feel. I created T-Tapp to do more than just burn calories and fat. This workout also helps the body rebuild primary body functions—such as neurokinetic flow, resting glucose utilization rate, and lymphatic function (more on all this later)—enabling you to enjoy positive changes in digestion, assimilation, elimination, and mental clarity right away.

By centering on your body's core—the area around your trunk and pelvis—T-Tapp builds muscles that cinch, uplift, tighten, and tone your body. With T-Tapp, you don't have to worry about developing the short, bulky muscles commonly associated with weight lifting. Instead, T-Tapp builds long, lean, sculpted muscles. This type of muscle development results in rapid inch loss. In fact, with T-Tapp, most people lose inches every single week they work out.

T-Tapp doesn't require a huge investment of your time, either. With this program, I'm going to show you fitness shortcuts you'll love. I'm also going to teach you how to work smarter, not harder, as well as how to maximize your muscle development and inch loss. You can actually expect to lose inches two to three times faster with T-Tapp than with any other workout you've tried.

Since launching T-Tapp twenty-five years ago, "Yes you can!" has been my signature mantra. I say it often while leading workout sessions, speaking at seminars, and on my fitness videos. Now, in this book, I'm using it to promise that . . .

YES YOU CAN

Look better, feel better, and lose six to eight inches—or a clothing size—in just two weeks

Most traditional exercises are isotonic, meaning they work only part of the muscle instead of the full length of the muscle. To see what I mean, stop reading for a second and do a traditional biceps curl. As you tighten your muscles when you curl up and again when you uncurl, you feel it in the middle of the biceps, right? That's an example of an isotonic exercise. Adding hand weights to a biceps curl is what enables muscle fibers to shorten and thicken, which is what creates the traditional bulging biceps.

Now do a T-Tapp biceps curl. Place your fist on your shoulder and bring your elbow up to shoulder level, *making sure the elbow is behind the ear.* Keep push-

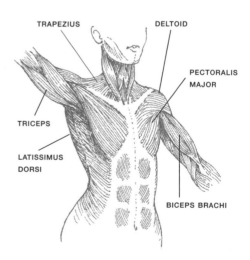

ing your elbow back to be in alignment with your shoulder. Now tighten as you curl and uncurl, but don't drop the elbow. In addition to the biceps, can you feel the triceps underneath? Can you also feel the deltoid muscles (or delts, shoulder muscles), as well as the latissimus dorsi (lats, the lateral muscles of the back) and the trapezius (traps, or back muscles)? *That's* the T-Tapp difference! You're working five muscles, full fiber, from the shoulder to the elbow, instead of one muscle just from the elbow to the belly of the muscle. And that's why in addition to building long, lean, sculpted muscles, you never have to do more than eight repetitions of any T-Tapp exercise to get results.

Margie Weiss

A magazine cover girl at age fifty!

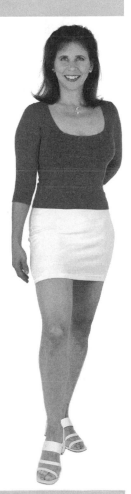

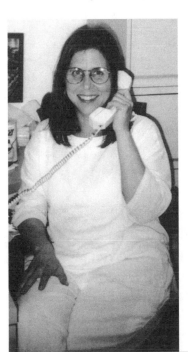

At forty-eight, it was harder for me to lose weight. Being a single mom of a teenage daughter and owning my own business left little time for me. But I could do the T-Tapp workout at home, and I got results fast. In fact, I lost a clothing size in the first two weeks! Over the next four months, I transformed myself from a middle-age 40-30-42-inch figure to a sexy 37-27-37-inch figure, which landed me on the cover of Woman's World *magazine in August 2001! Now it's easy to maintain my shape with just two workouts a week.*

With every T-Tapp move, you use the full length of your muscles, plus you move multiple muscles at once. In fact, *every T-Tapp exercise* works five to seven muscles simultaneously, layer by layer from the inside out. That's what I mean by *comprehensive, compound muscle movement*. Even muscles that aren't attached to bones are activated by T-Tapp techniques to pull inward and upward, creating an internal tension that literally "sucks" you in. As a result, inch loss comes quickly—an average of one clothing size every two to four weeks, based on your individual fitness level.

YES YOU CAN

Get a flat belly without doing a single crunch

If you've ever done bunches of crunches yet still had a poochy belly, here's one reason why. Traditional crunches focus mainly on the upper abs, the region just above your belly button. That leaves out three portions that make up your midsection: lower abs, obliques, and transverse abs. However, when you work out using the T-Tapp stance—shoulders back, butt tucked, and knees bent with KLT (knees pushing out to the little toes)—every single movement in the workout engages every single muscle within the abdominal area.

REAL PEOPLE, REAL RESULTS

Debra Shafer

"My tummy looked as if it had melted right off!"

When I first started T-Tapp, I had put on fifteen pounds in just a few weeks— extra weight that seemed to be hormone-related and surfaced mainly in my tummy area. This was the dangerous fat we women are warned about, and since I was approaching forty-three, I was concerned. I was also experiencing all of the serious symptoms of insulin resistance syndrome (IRS), a precursor to type 2 di-

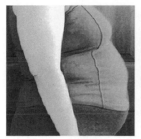 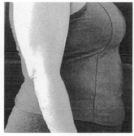 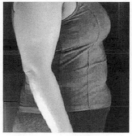 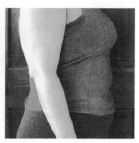

| STARTING | 2 WEEK | 60 DAY | 90 DAY |

abetes, which runs in my family. Because of this, coupled with being tired all the time and various aches and pains—especially in my knees—I felt I was headed down the path of serious health troubles.

After two weeks of T-Tapping, my tummy looked as if it had melted right off! Even more surprising, the brown velvety patches under my breasts (also symptoms of IRS), which had been present for two years, completely disappeared. I'm sure it was due to the regulating of my blood sugar levels and hormones from T-Tapp, as I hadn't made any other major changes. I also lost six pounds and a whopping thirteen and a half inches. As my strength increased, so did my energy levels, and I soon realized that I no longer had any aches or pains.

After that fourteen-day boot camp, I switched to working out three to five days a week. At the end of sixty days, I was twenty-two inches and two sizes smaller. My alignment and posture have improved dramatically, mostly due to dropping that tummy weight. I feel like a winner!

What's more, T-Tapp's full-fiber activation of muscle tissue can uplift, cinch, tighten, and tone abdominal muscles like never before. I often explain this "girdle effect" on muscles by remarking how men can instantly suck in their guts by six inches or more when a pretty girl walks by. That's the muscles pulling the abdominal organs in. And that's what T-Tapp moves can do for you—permanently.

When you stand up straighter or suck your tummy in, your belly instantly appears flatter. But there's no comparable technique you can use to suck in back fat. Back fat is a phenomenon that often plagues people age thirty and over, regardless of activity level. I often call this "fat shift" a reflection of internal core density. As your posture becomes less straight, the spinal muscle attachments become less active—or even inactive, depending on how poor your posture is. Active muscle tissue prefers fat for fuel, and excess glucose in the body converts to fat. But since these posture muscles aren't being activated, less fuel (both glucose and fat) is needed. Thus, back fat starts to accumulate.

REAL PEOPLE, REAL RESULTS

Bekki Johnson

Bye-bye back fat—and much, much more!

My journey with T-Tapp began in January 2002. My daughter had just celebrated her first birthday, and I had yet to lose any of the weight from my pregnancy. In fact, I may have been even heavier than the day after delivery. The extra weight showed everywhere but was particularly noticeable on my back, and I had no clue how to get rid of that

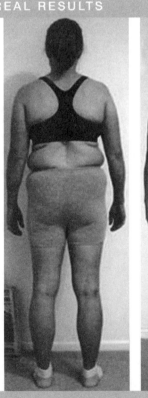
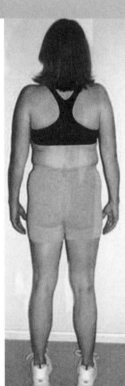

flab! When I heard about T-Tapp, I researched it online for a few weeks and then decided to try it.

By the fall of 2002, I had reached my ideal clothing size. It felt wonderful! In January 2003, I got pregnant with my fourth child. After the morning sickness subsided, I worked out by walking and doing all of the standing T-Tapp moves. I T-Tapped up until the day my second daughter was born.

Fast-forward to August 2004. Not only is the back fat gone, but in two months, I lost more than twenty inches and nine pounds. I started out wearing a size fourteen, and now I'm fitting comfortably into my size ten clothes. I can even button the eights, but they are still a bit too tight. Thank you for "the workout that works!"

The good news: T-Tapp burns back fat faster than any other workout currently on the market. That's because the comprehensive, compound movements in this workout activate all those postural muscles—layer by layer, from the inside out.

YES YOU CAN

Fire up your sluggish metabolism by building more calorie-hungry muscle

T-Tapp exercises are designed to stimulate the body to use glucose as fuel to support muscle movement instead of storing glucose as fat. Muscles are more metabolically active than other body tissue, meaning they are little calorie-burning machines. In fact, studies show that every pound of muscle you add increases your metabolism by thirty-five to fifty calories per day.

Traditional exercises build, at most, five pounds of muscle in a month or two. T-Tapp builds internal core muscles faster—*up to five to seven pounds in as little as one week!* So, in essence, you can raise your calorie-burning power by as much as 350 calories per day without any change in diet.

Increasing your muscle density is like increasing the size of the engine in your car. Everyone knows that larger engines require more fuel (calories) while idling (resting) as well as while cruising down the highway (exercising). So, by building more muscle, you not only gain the strength to work harder when exercising, but also enjoy the benefits of "afterburn." In other words, you condition your metabolism to continue torching calories even when you're at rest.

Worried about bulking up and resembling the Incredible Hulk? Don't be. Pound for pound, muscle takes up about 30 percent less space than fat, and unlike fat cells—which continue to expand as they grow—muscle tissue becomes more dense. With T-Tapp, you're also working muscles at both ends, so you don't have to worry about bulking up muscles in the middle. Instead, your muscles will get long and lean—and your body will get firm and slim.

YES YOU CAN

Maintain stronger bones without lifting a single weight

As you age, bones become less solid and less dense. This can eventually lead to osteoporosis, a disease in which your bones become more fragile and are more likely to break. Once thought to be a disease solely affecting postmenopausal women, osteoporosis is now known to affect younger women and even men.

While aerobic exercises offer many excellent health benefits, not all of them make your bones stronger. Strength training does this best. For example, in a yearlong study of postmenopausal women conducted at Tufts University, lifting weights just two days a week resulted in a 1 percent gain in hip and spinal density, a 13 percent increase in dynamic balance, and a 75 percent increase in overall strength and endurance.

Berei Brandenstein

She's standing taller with T-Tapp

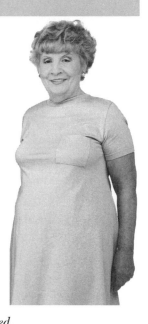

I was seventy-three when I first met Teresa Tapp at a free seminar. When I heard her saying that anyone could do her fitness program—the youngest T-Tapper at the time was nine, and the oldest was sixty—I remember wondering, "Does that 'anyone' include me?"

At the end of the seminar, I rushed up to Teresa and asked if she thought I would be able to do the exercises. She invited me to work out with her the next morning and was quite impressed that I did the exercises pretty well for my first time. Of course, my form needed correcting, but I was hooked.

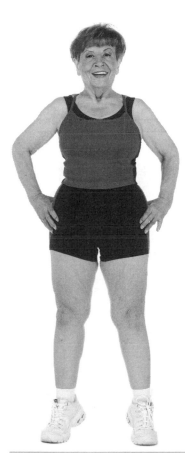

When I started T-Tapping, I was five feet one and a half inches tall and weighed 158 pounds. I had a dowager's hump and severe osteoporosis. I was on blood pressure, cholesterol, and osteoporosis medications. Now, at age seventy-eight, I have lost a total of fifty-two inches and twenty-five pounds. I'm also standing much straighter, having gained an inch in height, 20 percent more bone density in my right shoulder, and 7 percent more bone density in my lower lumbar area. I'm happy to say that I am also off all my medications. In fact, my doctor was so impressed with my well-being that he said he'd better start T-Tapping!

I have participated in many exercise programs, from water aerobics and weight training to tai chi, Pilates, and yoga—but I've never had the energy or the overall good feeling that I've enjoyed with T-Tapp . . . not to mention the phenomenal results. And the best part is that I did all this without dieting!

However, done improperly, weight training can create muscle imbalance, where certain muscles get stronger than others. Not only does that offset the better bone benefits, it also increases your chances of injury. That's why I teach you how to use your body as the machine—to create its own weight resistance with muscle movement.

Another problem with traditional strength training workouts is that not only do you have to go to a gym or buy specialized equipment, you also have to continue to add weight or do more repetitions to get results. But not with T-Tapp. Again, this workout positions your body in such a way that you use your muscles as the machine and create your own resistance. Thus, you simply don't need weights to get results. What's more, this technique forces your muscles to tighten and tug on the bones they're attached to, so you not only prevent osteoporosis by strengthening existing bones, but also stimulate new bone growth. In fact, it's never too early or too late to build better bones with T-Tapp.

Traditional weight training exercises build strength, but T-Tapp techniques build strength *and* flexibility, particularly in your core muscles. Why is this important? A strong, flexible core better equips you to handle the physical activities of daily living—like carrying groceries, lifting children, or just getting out of a chair—with greater ease and fewer aches and pains. That's why T-Tapp is known as the ultimate functional fitness workout.

With T-Tapp, you can reap all these bone-building benefits without ever worrying about adding more weight or doing more than eight repetitions. That's because T-Tapp moves continue to challenge your body even as your fitness level soars. In other words, the more you T-Tapp, the stronger you get—and the less you have to do it to maintain results.

Cardiac rehabilitative nurse and certified clinical exercise specialist Lannette Madden, R.N., agrees: "Since I started T-Tapping, I can bench-press more than when I was lifting super-heavy weights!"

Carbohydrates are *not* the enemy; in fact, they are absolutely necessary for cellular energy. Granted, the body does use carbohydrates to make blood sugar, and excess glucose can aggressively promote the accumulation of body fat. So the trick to eating carbohydrates and staying trim lies in helping the body use glucose *before* it's converted to fat.

Although the T-Tapp workout enables the body to do that already, sometimes you need a faster fix to burn that glucose. There's a little move within my workout called Hoe Downs that can allow you to eat, cheat, and get away with it. This move can be done alone and has been proven to help the body drop glucose levels an average of 62 to 85 points within three minutes. That's faster than an insulin shot!

Hoe Downs have been used to manage diabetic conditions; in fact, many T-Tappers with type 2 or gestational diabetes have regained control—and even reversed the disease—within three to six months.

REAL PEOPLE, REAL RESULTS

Denise Hentze

"Just call me 'the little engine that could'!"

I was practically born addicted to sugar, chocolate, cheese, and carbs. Of course, living in New Orleans didn't help matters. I could eat a half dozen beignets covered with powdered sugar at a sitting, along with bread pudding with tons of sauce. Jambalaya, gumbo, French bread and butter—my oh my, I could go on and on.

Over the years, I lost weight, but beginning in 1988, when my fiancé died suddenly, I regained it all—and then some. My doctor also prescribed antidepressants, and those made me gain even more. By 1999, I looked like a football player in a dress—no neck, couldn't see my feet, size twenty-four jeans—and I was on seventeen different medications!

I started T-Tapping in January 2000. Just doing the exercises—no dieting—I was into a size twelve by year's end, despite taking off two months in the summer. I lost a total of seventy-one inches, and I'm only fifty-nine inches tall (four feet eleven inches).

Recently I turned fifty, and I'm in control of my life, my health, and where I'm going. Now I'm only on four medications. In short, I am one happy camper!

How can Hoe Downs lower blood sugar so fast? To help you better understand this, let me share the results of some recent research conducted by Heinz Drexel, M.D., at the Voralberg Institute in Feldirch, Austria. His study took forty-five healthy but sedentary people and had them hike either up or down a steep mountain in the Austrian Alps each day for two months, then switch for another two months. Thirty-six hours after each hike, subjects' blood sugar, cholesterol, and triglycerides were checked. Results? It was no surprise that walking uphill lowered triglycerides, which are important components of cholesterol, but even Dr. Drexel was surprised to learn that downhill walkers exhibited a lowering of blood sugar levels not seen by those hiking only uphill.

These results make perfect sense to me. Think about your typical posture when walking downhill. You lean back and your shoulders and hips are in alignment, right? Well, that's the same posture used in the T-Tapp workout.

Hoe Downs are also perfect for burning off excess glucose after eating a high-carb meal or snack. I've heard lots of stories of T-Tappers running into bathrooms at restaurants and movie theaters to do a quick set of Hoe Downs to burn off the buttered popcorn or high-carb meal they have just consumed *before* it hits their saddlebags, belly, or butt!

Additionally, you can use Hoe Downs anytime you need an extra boost of energy or crave clarity of mind. I frequently rely on Hoe Downs to prevent that dreaded midafternoon slump. Although it looks simple, you'll be surprised at how aerobically challenging and invigorating this little move is.

YES YOU CAN

Avoid the middle-age spread commonly associated with menopause

Most women (and many men) can relate to the ongoing battle against increasing fat that seems to begin in our twenties, accelerates in our thirties, accumulates in our forties, and explodes in our fifties. Even though we may consume the same amount of calories and maintain the same level of exercise or activity, we seem to lose control over the formation of new fat.

Initially, this fat appears to shift to new areas of concern. Suddenly our bodies develop thunder thighs, bra pudge, back fat, or saddlebags. But eventually this excess fat seems to make its way to the abdominal area and cover hard-earned muscle tissue. The commonsense approach to getting rid of this "Buddha belly" is to reduce calories and increase exercise. While this may work initially, eventually the fat wins. What to do? Center on the core!

I first studied the relationship of hormones, insulin, and metabolism in females over age thirty when I was in college. Based on my own research and what I've subsequently read and learned, I believe that spinal muscle density—the thickness of the muscles that attach to the spine—is one of the primary secrets to success when it comes to avoiding the middle-age spread associated with menopause, and here's why.

Involuntary muscle movement—the motion of the muscles that attach to the spine and enable us to stand upright, as well as that of the muscles involved in breathing—uses glucose for fuel. Active muscle movement, on the other hand, prefers fat for fuel. Because we use our arms and legs daily, we generally maintain muscle in those areas, but the majority of adults don't ride skateboards or do cartwheels, somersaults, or other movements that involve balance on a daily basis. Not to say that going upside down is required, but tilting, twisting, and rolling your spine is necessary to challenge your core muscles, and most adults' daily activity doesn't involve these kinds of movements.

What happens when we don't use these muscles involved in balance? We lose internal muscle tone, and atrophy begins. In fact, a decrease in spinal muscle density means less fuel (glucose) is needed for spinal support to maintain an upright position, so excess glucose starts to accumulate and gets converted to fat. But there's good news for T-Tappers: once glucose is expended—via exercises that strengthen the core—fat burning does occur.

To complicate matters even further, female hormones are almost always fluctuating. Our bodies are in a constant state of homeostasis— meaning each time our levels of estrogen increase, the pancreas reacts by releasing more insulin to help the body maintain hormonal balance. The problem is, insulin is considered to be a fat-producing hormone, meaning that it causes our body to store more fat. And unfortunately, if fat cells are already full, your body makes more fat cells—which is why I call this the vicious fat cycle. Incidentally, fat cells never disappear . . . they're always either empty or full.

Increased insulin produced in reaction to carbohydrate consumption can also increase estrogen levels. This in turn can cause even more insulin to be produced. To make matters worse, women undergo additional hormonal changes—particularly excess estrogen in comparison to progesterone (estrogen dominance)—during the onset of menopause. The result? Female fat accumulation continues to grow with increased furor as we age—*unless* we maintain or rebuild our resting glucose utilization rate.

Angela Flores

"My hormones are finally stable!"

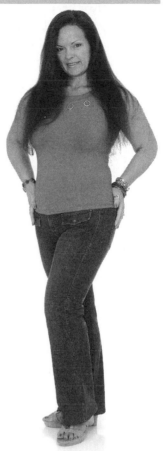

At age twenty-nine, I had a hysterectomy, which left my hormones in a state of chaos and packed on the pounds. For twenty-five years, I've also suffered with a case of chronic fibrocystic breasts. My marriage suffered, because I could not stand for my husband to touch me. It hurt to walk or wear a bra. When I had mammograms, the radiologist would always find something suspicious because the cysts made up most of my breast tissue.

With T-Tapp, I found almost instant relief. In two months, I noticed a greater stabilization in my body and hormone levels. The breast pain was gone. I had no swelling. My body was also trimmer. I could see my ankle bones, and my abdomen was flatter. I noticed definition in my torso, and the cellulite on my thighs was greatly diminished. I had even lost my third butt cheek (although I don't miss it), and my saddlebags were gone as well.

I went to the doctor a few months ago—the same breast surgeon I have been going to for years. He put my films up on the display light and did a double-take. "What did you do?" he asked. He could not believe the change in my breast tissue from one year to the next! And just a few days ago, I got my most recent mammogram results. For the first time in fifteen years, I had a normal report. I think I'll frame it!

Not sure what resting glucose utilization rate is? Similar to, but not quite the same as, basal metabolic rate, it's a process that enables your body to burn glucose at a premium—even when you're not moving. To get to that point, however, you need to maintain or rebuild muscle density on the spine, because it's those core muscles that prefer glucose for fuel to stand upright against gravity. To achieve that core density, spinal muscles need to be activated at both points of attachment for full fiber contraction. Remember, most traditional exercises are isotonic in nature, meaning that they activate only one muscle attachment. In contrast, T-Tapp moves are both *comprehensive,* meaning that they use both attachments of a muscle, and *compound,* meaning that they involve using multiple muscles at once. As a result, spinal muscle density increases, and the body becomes a virtual glucose furnace, even at rest— all of which helps to counter the weight gain commonly associated with menopause.

YES YOU CAN

Help your blood sugar stay in check

Roller-coaster blood sugar levels cause a lot of fattening side effects, including hunger pangs, food cravings, and fatigue. Whenever you have too much blood sugar (glucose) circulating in your system, your body tries to balance it by releasing more insulin, which is known as the fat-producing hormone. But with T-Tapp, you're working core and large muscles at the same time, which burns glucose super-fast to keep insulin levels down—plus T-Tapp builds muscle density along the spine, and those core muscles are primarily the ones that burn glucose for fuel, even at rest. So, in simple terms, by maintaining better core muscle density, you're helping your body help itself maintain a better balance of blood sugar. This, in turn, helps your body to prevent fat storage from occurring due to excess sugar in the blood.

Aimee Dubuisson

She's the Hoe Down queen!

Two years ago, I was diagnosed with severe type 2 diabetes. I was dehydrated, obese, and sicker than I'd ever been in my life. Walking to the kitchen for a glass of water was a major chore and caused me shortness of breath and chest pains.

I was already taking two different kinds of diabetes medications, but my blood sugar consistently stayed in the 350–400 range [80–120 is normal]. My doctor recommended an insulin pump as a last resort. That meant submitting to this disease, and I wasn't ready for that—at least not emotionally. So I asked my doctor to give me a little more time on the medication to see if it would by some miracle kick in. He gave me two weeks.

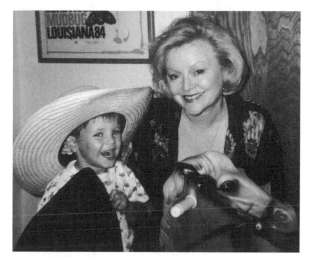

The next day, I heard Teresa Tapp on a morning radio show. She was offering a free seminar, and I couldn't wait to attend. Walking from the parking lot to the hotel meeting room was almost more than I could bear, but everything Teresa said made sense. Suddenly, I felt hopeful.

I started T-Tapping the next day, and within ten days I had lost ten inches. But that's not what I was most excited about. A mere four days into the workout, my blood sugar began to respond. In fact, after those first ten days, my doctor had to reduce both my diabetes and heart medications! Two months later, he discontinued all my medications, and I've had perfectly normal blood sugar levels ever since! I continue to keep my blood sugar in check by doing Hoe Downs while making copies at the office.

Oh, by the way, I also lost twenty-five pounds and over twenty inches. I'm four feet eleven inches tall and have gone from a super-tight size fourteen to a size ten. I'm still losing and must say I look pretty darned cute for someone who is fifty-five years young!

When T-Tapping, your muscles work overtime in that you're not just doing isometric moves but simultaneously moving large muscles. This allows your body to kick into fat burning quicker. Best of all, the combination of having greater muscle density and doing T-Tapp causes your body to burn more fat while sabotaging its ability to *make* more fat.

YES YOU CAN

Banish back pain

Back pain has reached such epidemic proportions that it has become a fact of life for most people. Studies show it's one of the most common disorders for which people seek medical help, accounting for over 100 million lost work days each year—ranking ahead of fever, knee pain, rashes, and headaches. Back pain is also responsible for a whopping $97 billion in annual medical costs.

There have been many theories as to why and how back pain occurs. Medical science used to teach us that back pain was due to structural abnormalities or misalignment of the spine, but now a lot of other factors are being considered. We've come to realize, for example, that tension might be the cause of most back pain. In our busy, nonstop, stressful lives, we often forget to take a break and stretch.

As a rehabilitative trainer, I realize that tension causes muscles to tighten and blood vessels to constrict. Depending on how weak or how strong a person's muscles are, this tension can pull vertebrae out of alignment and reduce blood flow. Of course, it doesn't help matters that the majority of women today wear high heels, cross their legs for long periods of time, and often stand with their weight on one leg while holding the telephone between ear and shoulder or a child on one hip. No wonder our back and shoulder muscles hurt by the end of the day!

Marion Coleman

"The chiropractor can wait!"

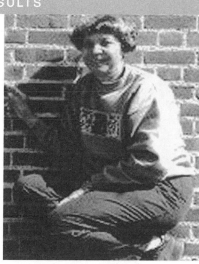

When I first heard about T-Tapp on WPVI-TV in Philadelphia, I was a size sixteen and not happy with the way I looked. I didn't feel that great, either—my back hurt a lot, and I was having arthritis pains in my knee.

I've always walked in the morning for about forty minutes and continue to do so. But now after walking, I do T-Tapp for about thirty-five minutes every other day. Most evenings I also do Primary Back Stretch, Organs in Place/Half Frogs, or some other T-Tapp move. As a result, I've lost forty-three inches and eighteen pounds—with no dieting.

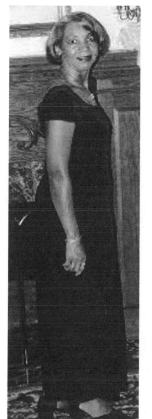

I am currently down to a very comfortable size twelve and feel better than I have in years. I'm so much stronger, and my arms have that "cut" look without even using weights. I still have a chiropractor's card in my wallet to remind me that I was supposed to make an appointment. No need for that now! Once I started T-Tapping, I have not had any back problems, and the arthritis in my knee has really improved. In fact, I recently walked in the Philadelphia Marathon! My time was 5 hours 54 minutes for the 26.2-mile walk. This year, I am training to walk the Marine Corps Marathon in Washington, D.C. Without T-Tapp, I would never have been able to get into shape, nor have the confidence to attempt a marathon.

One of the reasons I've been so successful as a rehabilitative trainer is because I know and understand how back pain feels due to my own spinal condition. As I explained in Chapter 1, I suffer from scoliosis, a slight curvature of the spine, along with fusion of three lumbar vertebrae resulting from a high school sports injury. In addition, my psoas muscles often lock into spasms and pull on these three vertebrae. Due to these issues, if I don't keep my spinal muscles strong and flexible with T-Tapp, my back hurts!

Let me tell you, pain is a great teacher. When developing the T-Tapp workout, I focused on creating exercises that would help stretch and strengthen spinal muscles, increase blood flow, and deliver relief from chronic back pain. It works for me, and if you suffer from back pain, it will work for you, too.

YES YOU CAN

Improve your posture as you reshape your body

T-Tapp centers on the spine—not just for core muscle development but also for better spinal alignment. This lessens the chance of injury that often increases with age, plus pulls everything in toward your spine. As a result, not only do you tighten muscles, you also lengthen them. And when that happens, you stand up straighter without even thinking about it. Check the mirror, and you'll quickly discover that good posture makes you look thinner—instantly. It also enables you to project an air of confidence.

T-Tapp offers even more benefits in terms of posture, particularly as you age. "When you think of an elderly person, you usually conjure up a vision of someone stooped over with rounded shoulders and shuffling along—often with a cane," notes Lannette Madden. "But guess what? This posture doesn't just happen overnight. It's set into motion when you are still young and then cascades as you get older." Fortunately, T-Tapp not only breaks this cycle, but also can reverse it—and it's never too late to do so.

Indeed, one of Madden's clients recently left her T-Tapp class but came back in the door a few minutes later. "When I asked why he was back, he told me he had forgotten his cane and hadn't realized it until he got outside!" she reports.

Not only does T-Tapp improve your posture, it strengthens your pectoral muscles, which, in essence, gives you a mini breast lift. In fact, with this workout, you can get perkier pecs, regardless of cup size! How so? As we age, many female bodies suffer from a gravitational pulling down of the chest. But since T-Tapp moves involve pulling the shoulders back into better alignment, this in turn pulls the bosom up—plus tightens and tones those pecs.

REAL PEOPLE, REAL RESULTS

Lucy Johnson

With T-Tapp, she got perkier pecs!

T-Tapp has improved my posture, eliminated my lower back pain, made me more flexible, and helped me lose inches. I was particularly impressed with how much I lost within the first two weeks.

I received my college degree in microbiology, and the research that Teresa has done and the explanations and studies done to support the science behind the exercises make so much sense to me. I still have more to lose, but I now know that I am capable of completing my goal and that I am on my

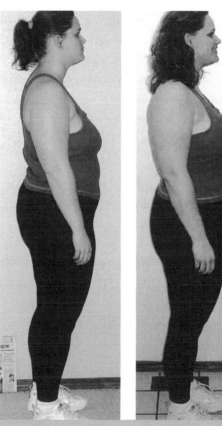

way to achieving the body and health that I deserve. Best of all, my children are now used to seeing their mother exercise, and I love *knowing that I am setting a great example for them.*

With most exercises, you have to sweat for twenty minutes to get into fat-burning mode, but with T-Tapp, this process can take as little as ten minutes. You can chalk this advantage up to T-Tapp's ability to turbocharge glucose metabolism in the body. But there's more at work here. T-Tapp also promotes neurokinetic flow, or greater nerve transmission from the brain through the spine to the extremities. Let me explain.

With T-Tapp, almost every move is performed with shoulders back and aligned with the hips, butt tucked, knees bent, and KLT (knees pushing toward the little toes). This stance properly aligns your spine, so nerve transmissions can clearly make their way to your extremities.

REAL PEOPLE, REAL RESULTS

Stephanie Ackerman

"I can now wear the jeans I've always dreamed of wearing!"

I started gaining weight as a teen and really put it on in college. I spent my twenties losing and gaining and going through a vicious cycle of dieting and rebounding. During my second pregnancy, I gained over seventy pounds on a diet of powdered sugar doughnuts and Pepperidge Farm Sausalito cookies. I was huge! Over seven years, I faithfully went to the gym, did karate, played tennis, bought many exercise tapes, and used the treadmill. I lost sixty-five pounds, but I was not satisfied with the way I looked and felt.

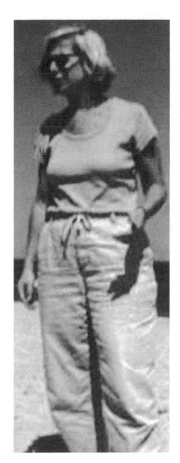

My goal was to find a way-of-life fitness program by my fortieth birthday, and T-Tapp was the answer. The first time I did the workout, I was hooked. Not only have I lost inches, but my body has noticeably changed. I don't look bulky; I look trim and toned. My shape is more defined and curvy. My waist, hips, and thighs are more in proportion. I can now wear the jeans that I have always dreamed of wearing.

T-Tapp has allowed me to stay strong and healthy— I haven't had a major cold in two winters. My hormones are better balanced as well. Before starting T-Tapp, I was scheduled to have surgery due to excessive bleeding with my menstrual cycle. After one month of T-Tapp, however, my cycle returned to normal!

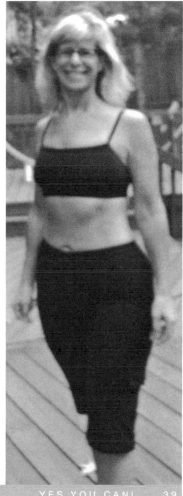

T-Tapp has taught me what an amazing piece of equipment my body is. It has given me confidence and a brighter outlook towards aging and my health. I truly feel that I'm not getting older, just better!

Why is this important? For starters, if muscles don't receive full nerve stimulus, they can't possibly perform at peak levels. Nerve transmission is what makes muscles move, so better nerve transmission results in a higher metabolism, more efficient muscle activity, faster inch and weight loss, and higher energy levels.

Sounds a bit complicated, I know, but think of neurokinetic flow as being similar to unkinking a garden hose. When you water the flowers with a kinked hose, you're still watering them, but it's not nearly as effective because you're not getting enough water pressure. But when you unkink the hose, everything flows faster and you get the job done in half the time.

YES YOU CAN

Boost your immune system so you rarely get sick

Most traditional exercise programs focus on burning calories and losing weight, whereas T-Tapp focuses on building a better lymphatic system and losing inches. Having a well-functioning lymphatic system is crucial for overall health and well-being because it supports the immune system. That's why people with autoimmune diseases such as chronic fatigue, lupus, or fibromyalgia report great benefits from T-Tapp. It's also why cancer patients undergoing radiation or chemotherapy who practice T-Tapp have fewer side effects. And it's precisely why those who T-Tapp don't seem to get sick as often.

A healthy lymphatic system has been found to be particularly beneficial for people with autoimmune diseases. In this area, a recent monthlong study conducted at the Veterans Administration Hospital in New Port Richey, Florida, turned up some impressive diagnostic results after just eight sessions of T-Tapp. In addition to an average loss of eight and a half inches, there were noticeable reductions in severity of chronic medical problems, as measured by blood pressure, cholesterol levels, symptoms, and overall feelings of well-being.

Naomi Armstrong

"For me, T-Tapp was the best medicine!"

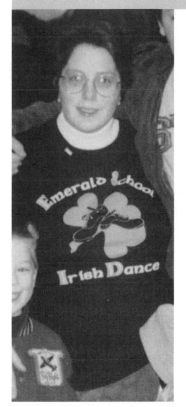

Six years ago, I was diagnosed with systemic lupus and fibromyalgia. I tried a variety of medications and finally found a combination that worked best for me, but I was still in a lot of pain. I consistently had a tingling feeling in my hands and feet and couldn't sense temperatures unless they were extreme. I used a walker for two and half months and a cane for probably another three months after that. I worried about how long I'd be able to work and about keeping up with my young children. Plus, the medications had driven my weight and clothing size way up.

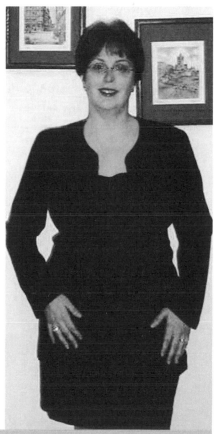

My doctors said that exercising would help with the pain, so I tried aerobics, dancing, running, walking, and weight lifting. Nothing seemed to make any difference. I was still having very high levels of pain.

Then I found T-Tapp. After just a few days, my pain was gone! I was also excited to drop several dress sizes. To me, the inch loss was icing on the cake; I will keep T-Tapping for life because of the pain relief.

Prior to T-Tapping, I had consulted with two different neurologists. Both told me I had seen all the improvement I would ever see. Boy, were they wrong! T-Tapp has increased my endurance, my balance is better, and I've regained feeling in my hands and feet. Plus, I haven't taken a prescription pain pill since October 2002! This is truly a program I can see myself doing for life.

There were inspiring anecdotal successes as well. For example, one VA receptionist who had suffered from chronic fatigue syndrome for five years reported, "I used to be so exhausted that I couldn't do anything after I got home from work. Now, after only thirty days of doing T-Tapp, I have so much energy. In fact, just last week, I mowed my lawn!"

Mention the heart or cardiovascular system, and most folks have a pretty good idea of what it is and how it functions. But although the lymphatic system is vitally important to your health and well-being, most people don't understand it. I'm quite familiar with it because of my own sluggish lymphatic system, which still results in a lump in my armpit. In fact, I was studying the lymphatic system back when it was still considered part of the circulatory system. So, let me give you the lowdown on what it is, how it works, and why it's so important.

The lymphatic system is a network of fluid-filled tubes that continuously bathes our cells and then carries away the body's "sewage"—toxins, waste products of metabolism, globules of fat, excess liquid—to filters called lymph nodes, where harmful substances are trapped and neutralized. In fact, there is three times more lymph fluid than there is blood in the body. But while blood has a pump—the heart—to keep it moving, lymph fluid must be pumped by the movement of our muscles. So the less we move, the more stagnant our lymph system becomes.

Many people have sluggish lymph systems and don't even know it. Swollen lymph glands, of course, are one telltale sign. But oftentimes allergies, chronic sinusitis, high blood pressure, loss of energy, arthritis, and even headaches can be attributed to blocked or congested lymph nodes!

What does pumping the lymphatic system have to do with our waistlines? Plenty. In fact, research reveals that as many as 80 percent of overweight women have sluggish lymphatic systems.

With the help of the circulatory system, the lymphatic system moves liquefied fats throughout the body, and since all T-Tapp moves pump the lymph system, you're circulating liquefied fats throughout the entire body. Since that liquefied fat is then used as fuel for your muscles, you become a greater fat-burning machine. What's more, fluids that accumulate can cause bloating—and bloated tissue can cause us to swell up to two extra clothing sizes. Bloated tissues also prevent cells from properly absorbing nutrients and oxygen. In a sense, the cells begin to starve. And as cells starve for nutrients, it only makes sense that intense hunger pangs and cravings will set in. Worse, without adequate oxygen to ignite the metabolic process, fewer calories are burned. Many scientists also believe that a lazy lymphatic system is directly connected to the formation of cellulite.

The good news is once you get your lymphatic system pumping at full force, your body becomes better equipped to eliminate toxins naturally in addition to providing more fuel for muscles—plus your junk food cravings will be drastically curbed. Bonus: in addition to a firm and toned body, a free-flowing lymphatic system also makes for clear, smooth, glowing skin. It literally helps your body help itself.

YES YOU CAN

Win the war against cellulite

Most of us are all too familiar with that unsightly dimpled tissue that ripples across the thighs, hips, and buttocks. Despite what you've heard—that cellulite is nothing more than ordinary fat—there's a lot more going on here. Cellulite involves trapped toxins, poor circulation, weaker muscles, and thinner skin—all of which cause the layer of fat beneath to clump like little blobs of Jell-O.

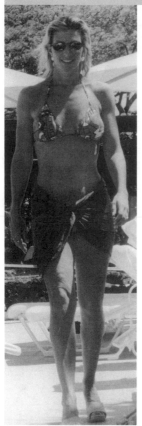

Erin Conway

Yes, you can get rid of the ripple effect!

I've always been an active person who loves fitness. I'm athletic, work out on a regular basis, and watch what I eat—so why did I have cellulite all over my thighs? Thankfully I found T-Tapp and learned how to help control cellulite from the inside out. Within weeks I lost inches, built muscle, and got my cellulite completely under control! T-Tapp really works!

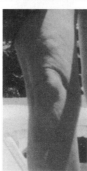

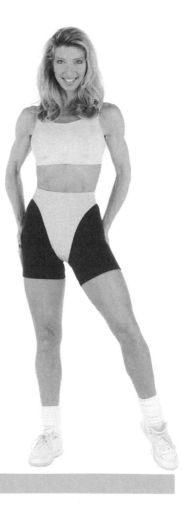

The good news is that T-Tapp exercises comprehensively battle the bumps. How? By building a better lymph system that eliminates trapped toxins; by rebuilding neurokinetic flow, which improves circulation (even to the point that most who T-Tapp no longer have cold hands or cold feet); and by developing muscles with girdle-like strength that not only burn fat but help smooth out the bumps. T-Tapp also helps control cellulite by promoting the importance of body brushing (see Appendix) to exercise the skin as well as the muscles.

YES YOU CAN

Get an energy makeover

Fatigue, particularly among women, accounts for close to fifteen million doctor visits every year. The best prescription for feeling run down? Get your body moving and your blood pumping! T-Tapp exercises may not *look* aerobic, but they will definitely raise your heart rate. And when that happens, your adrenaline level skyrockets, and you'll feel a definite energy boost!

REAL PEOPLE, REAL RESULTS

Meredith Decker

This mom now has energy to burn!

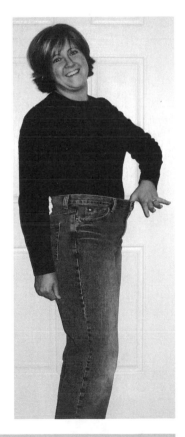

I'm everywoman! Okay, not everywoman, but I do represent a large population of thirty-something women with young children, who are slightly overweight and out of shape and who feel they don't have enough time or energy for themselves. At thirty-three, with three boys under the age of six, I can tell you that there are simply not enough hours in the day to accomplish everything that needs to be done. However, I can also tell you that T-Tapp is a great workout, with a very doable time commitment, and it delivers results.

I have lost ten and three-quarters inches and one pants size. My energy level is up, my mood swings have lessened dramatically, my skin is clear, my clothes fit better, and I feel good about myself. Do I have to add that a happy mommy leads to a happy family?

"Although the reasons aren't clear, T-Tapp also seems to increase the body's ability to clear lactic acid, which in turn seems to increase endurance," says Lannette Madden. "One marathon runner I coached shaved twenty minutes off her race time after T-Tapping for just four months!"

That doesn't surprise me. Lactic acid, a waste product of muscles, is what causes that "burning" sensation felt in your muscles during high-intensity exercise. It can prevent your muscles from working their best and can also make your body feel sore after a workout. But since the lymphatic system is one of your body's elimination systems, and T-Tapp exercises excel at pumping lymph, lactic acid doesn't accumulate in muscle tissue. Instead, it is released into the lymphatic system and carried away with each and every T-Tapp move.

YES YOU CAN

Boost your brainpower

With most traditional exercise programs, you work just one side of your body—and your brain—at a time. Right leg lifts, for example, followed by left leg lifts. But I designed T-Tapp to be a left-brain/right-brain, mind/body workout. For example, when you lift your right leg, the left side of your brain is in control. During T-Tapp moves, however, while the left side of your brain is focusing on keeping the right knee bent and pushing toward the little toe, the right side of your brain is simultaneously focusing on performing large muscle movements (leg lifts, for instance) on the left side of the body. Numerous neurological studies have shown that by working both sides of the brain at once, you stimulate the creation of new neural pathways between the right and left hemispheres of your brain. As a result, your learning ability, memory, intuition, and creativity improve—plus you're better able to focus, concentrate, and think more clearly. Whole-brain functioning, as scientists call it, is also important as we age, because it improves kinetic awareness, thus helping to prevent the clumsy trips and falls often associated with the elderly.

Many people think it's a given that mental capacities diminish with age. Not so, according to neurosurgeon Arthur Winter, M.D., co-author of *Brain Workout: Easy Ways to Power Up Your Memory, Sensory Perception and Intelligence*. His research has found that cognitive decline doesn't occur in *healthy* older brains. Basically, there are two keys to remaining super-sharp as we get older. The first is aerobic exercise, which counters the reduced oxygen levels in our blood as we age, which in turn can cause a decline in the neurotransmitters that allow brain cells to communicate with one another. "In one study, sedentary individuals ages 55 to 70 who enlisted in a four-month aerobic exercise program did significantly better on neuropsychology tests than those who didn't perform aerobic exercise," reports Dr. Winter. "And this improved cognitive performance was attributed to increased blood flow to the brain."

The second way to keep your noggin nourished as you age is to keep it stimulated. Contrary to popular belief, "your brain continues to repair cell damage and form new neural networks throughout life," Dr. Winter insists. "In fact, people who are active mentally can actually *improve* their performance on intelligence tests—even after age 60."

By T-Tapping, you're practically guaranteed a boost in brainpower—even as you get older. That's because T-Tapp exercises are aerobic as well as mentally stimulating.

YES YOU CAN

Retain your svelte shape with just three quickie workouts a week

With T-Tapp, the stronger you get, the more you get out of it—and the less you have to do it to stay in shape. In fact, once you reach your goal size, maintaining your figure requires T-Tapping just fifteen to forty-five minutes a day three times a week.

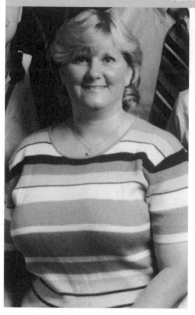

Carol Severson

She's the incredible shrinking woman!

I'm a forty-five-year-old mother of four who writes curriculum reviews for a national home-schooling catalog. I've also authored a book on home schooling. When I started T-Tapping, my schedule was jam-packed. Between home-school-ing my own children and traveling for speaking en-gagements on home schooling most weekends, I had packed a substantial amount of weight onto my originally tiny five-foot-one frame. Bursting out of a size fourteen and weighing 176 pounds, I was not happy when I looked in the mirror. Plus I was exhausted all the time.

When I first heard about T-Tapp, I was skeptical. In fact, I was convinced I was wasting time I didn't have. I was so wrong. Initially, I didn't dare weigh or measure myself, but after just one week, my clothes were feeling loose. After two weeks, I was down to a tight size ten—and extremely motivated to keep going.

By the end of three months, I had shrunk to a size eight (or a size six if I didn't want to take any deep breaths). Four weeks later, I was easily fitting into a size six and weighed 126 pounds.

I am now a slim 100 pounds, wearing a size zero—quite an accomplishment for someone who never, not even for a fraction of a second, believed this would work for me.

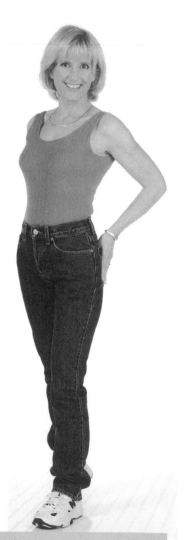

I still T-Tapp approximately every other day, but sometimes manage it just twice a week. I've learned that with T-Tapp, more is not always better. You don't need to do this workout every day to get great results!

How can this be? It's simple. The stronger you get, the more control you have over muscle contractions, so you can dig deeper and hold isometric contractions longer. In other words, you're maximizing your muscles more, so you're getting more out of each exercise. You're also building greater strength and flexibility, which enables you to maintain better body alignment for longer periods of time—and that maximizes your muscles' ability to cinch in.

Let's go back to the car analogy I used at the beginning of this chapter. After T-Tapping for a while, your body is literally a better-tuned machine. In fact, once it's tuned up and fully aligned, it can operate at full capacity with less effort.

Madden agrees. "I used to believe that if some exercise was good, more was better," she admits. "But T-Tapp has convinced me otherwise. I'm stronger and can run faster now than when I was working out ten to fifteen hours a week!"

Soon you'll believe it yourself. Why? Because by combining strength training (even though you'll never lift a dumbbell) and aerobics (no leaps or jumps required), as well as isometrics, balance training, and flexibility in one time-efficient package, less really *is* more with T-Tapp.

Getting Ready to T-Tapp

I know you think you're ready to flip to the next chapter and start the workout. I know you've probably tried many other exercise programs on the market and feel confident in your ability to do T-Tapp without a lot of background or instruction. And I also know that it's frustrating to keep reading about the *why* of everything instead of just getting down to doing it. But understanding form and learning how to do these exercises the right way is imperative if you're going to achieve rapid results. It's also critical to helping your body avoid injury. So keep reading, and you will learn how to align your body properly for T-Tapp, as well as how to master the all-important T-Tapp stance.

In this chapter, you'll also discover your body type and why it matters, plus you'll pick up plenty of pointers to help you create a personal workout schedule so you can achieve your desired results.

"Quit slouching!" "Stand up straight!" Growing up, how many times did you hear these phrases? Turns out your mom was right, but few of us actually stand correctly. Take a look at any anatomy or physiology textbook, and you'll see that the human body is positioned with arms at the sides and palms facing forward. This is considered correct anatomical position. Now take a look at your normal stance in the mirror. I'll bet that your palms automatically face backward. Although this stance is typical for most people, it can be problematic because it causes your shoulder joint to roll forward, which ultimately makes the upper spinal column curve forward. In fact, if you look closely, you'll probably notice a slight sloping from your neck to your shoulder—and depending on your age, you may already have some fat deposits there, at the base of your neck.

As we age, poor posture becomes more apparent and creates an imbalance in muscle strength—not only along the vertebrae and shoulder joints, but also in the compression of internal organs. It also creates an increased risk for back and/or shoulder injury—not to mention that compressed organs contribute to the development of lower abdominal pooch.

REAL PEOPLE, REAL RESULTS

Julyn Harrison

No more excuses!

Since T-Tapping over the last two months, I have gained so much. No, not in inches, but in so many valuable experiences. It is true that I have dropped fifteen inches, but what the inches mean emotionally and psychologically are even more important to me.

All my life I have used my weight as a protective shield. I always had an excuse not to look my best or prettiest. T-Tapp has given me the workable tools to address this part of my character. I've learned that it's exercising, not dieting, that will bring permanent changes. It's the kinetic awareness and the compound muscle movement. T-Tapp is about changing from the inside out. This workout has opened the door to that person that I had previously kept shut in a "prison" of fat and depression. I am so grateful!

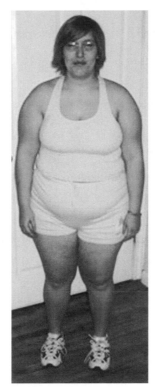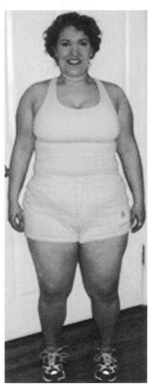

T-Tapp corrects all this by putting your knees, hips, spine, and shoulders into proper alignment—and that alone offers many benefits. For starters, it gives you better muscular balance and takes stress off your joints, allowing them to work together as nature intended. With proper alignment, your internal organs have room to function optimally, neural pathways are opened wide, and blood circulates more freely. What's more, abdominal muscles pull up in front and gluteal (buttocks) muscles pull down in back to maintain the spine's natural curve. This allows you to stay in a balanced standing posture for long periods of time without tiring.

With proper alignment, you avoid injury, because your muscles are developed in balance—so they build strength and flexibility equally. Best of all, proper alignment enables your muscles to work at maximum efficiency. How? Because now they're going to be used full fiber instead of isotonically, which means you'll be activating the full length of every muscle you move.

Getting your body into proper alignment is critical before you begin to T-Tapp. To do that, just find a mirror and . . .

ASSUME THE T-TAPP STANCE

Unless instructed otherwise, this is the position you should assume for every exercise in this book.

Step 1: Stand with feet hip width apart. Make sure that your ankles are planted directly beneath your hip joints. Your toes should be pointing forward, not turned out. Keep in mind that hip width apart is rarely as wide as people think it is. In fact, most new T-Tappers have a tendency to mistakenly place their feet shoulder width apart instead.

For proper placement, try this: Place your left foot forward and your right foot perpendicular to it with the heel of your right foot resting against the arch of your left foot. Now you need only pivot your right foot so that it's also facing forward. *This* is hip width apart.

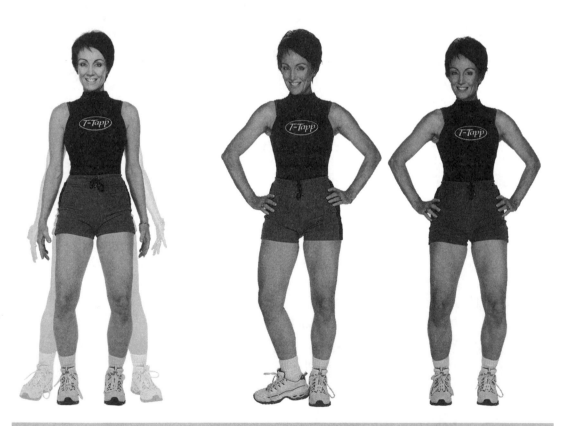

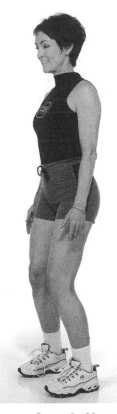

Step 2: Bend your knees. Feel how your muscles tighten just above the knees? Now straighten the knees. Feel how the thigh relaxes? Now bend the knees again and realize that the reason you're going to keep them bent at all times throughout the T-Tapp workout is so that you can maintain full fiber activation of all your leg muscles from the knee up. This helps you achieve optimal muscle density without building bulk.

How far to bend the knees? If you look down while in this position, you should not be able to see your feet. If you can see them, then you need to bend a little more. Another way to test yourself is to stand with your toes against a wall. Now bend your knees until they also touch the wall. This is how bent your knees should be throughout the entire T-Tapp workout. Your knees should be over your feet, aiming toward your little toes to the best of your ability.

Step 3: Now, keeping your knees bent, tuck your butt. This is more than just a tightening of the cheeks. Think along the lines of what a dog does when it's been caught being naughty. It tucks its tail between its legs. You should do the same—and tuck hard! Feel the muscles in your lower back as well as your tummy? When you tuck your butt, you get full fiber activation of the muscles that attach to your lower back (lower lumbar vertebrae), which crisscross to the opposite hip and create an abdominal girdle. This enables you to maintain a strong back and a flat stomach—without doing sit-ups!

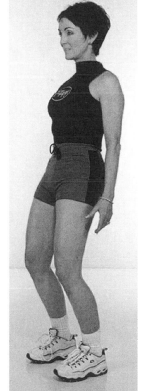

Step 4: Roll your shoulders back and down. Keep your knees bent and butt tucked, and align your shoulders with your hips, but do *not* arch your back! Do you feel

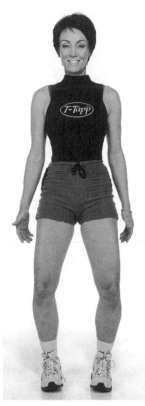

how your rib cage just lifted and your stomach pulled in? When your shoulders are back and aligned with the hips, this separates your ribs from your hips, so you have more room in your abdominal area. That means your muscles can cinch in and create a trimmer torso and a tighter tummy. It also activates more muscles in your back for spinal support.

Don't move—you're not done yet. Hold this position and move to Step 5.

Step 5: Push your knees out toward your little toes. This last step is what's known as KLT. Did you feel the lower tummy tighten? That's because you've just created full fiber activation of the transverse abdominal muscles, which helps you maintain a stronger pelvic floor and helps banish lower belly pooch. For men, the KLT position also helps to strengthen muscle attachments at the groin, which helps maintain a flatter lower belly and may even help prevent beer belly.

Keep in mind that KLT is more than just pointing your knees toward your little toes; it means rotating or turning your knees out from the hip socket. Doing this helps to create tighter muscle tension on the thigh muscles, leading to a beautiful shape.

By now, you might feel like you're riding on a horse. Don't worry—you're almost done. Stop for a minute and shake out your legs, then resume the T-Tapp stance (feet hip width apart with toes forward, knees bent, butt tucked, shoulders back, and KLT) and focus on your shoulders. With your arms resting along the sides of your body, do two shoulder rolls (lift shoulders up, back, and down in a circular motion), and pay attention to what muscles are being used.

THE T-TAPP STANCE

A quick reference

1. **Stand with feet hip width apart**

2. **Bend knees**

3. **Tuck butt**

4. **Pull shoulders back and down**

5. **Push knees out toward little toes (KLT)**

Now let's do the same movement the T-Tapp way. Flip your palms forward, stretch your fingers wide, and twist your thumbs to the wall behind you as far as you can. Do you feel the difference? Do you feel how every muscle in your upper back is activated? Now do four shoulder rolls in this position. By the third one, you may hear some snap, crackle, and pop. Don't worry—that's just natural chiropractic alignment of your upper back, with the muscles pulling on the cervical vertebrae for optimal spinal alignment and full fiber activation of your back muscles.

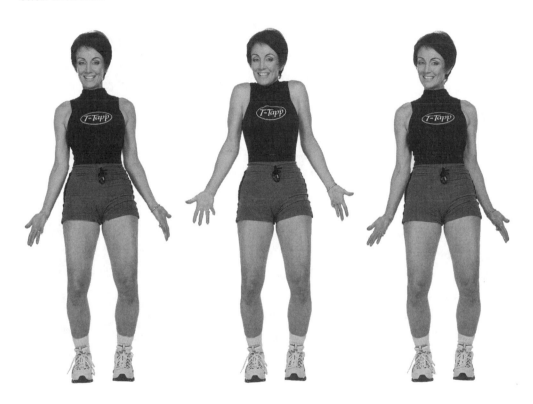

Pat Van Horn

"My 'fat' clothes are now in paper bags!"

I've been T-Tapping for a little over two years, am seventy years young, and have lost a total of forty-five inches and forty pounds. In addition to that good news, my cholesterol has come down. My gynecologist recently did a bone density test and found that my hip density, which had been at −2.2, was now at −1.1.

That's a 50 percent improvement in bone density! He asked what I'd been doing, and I told him all about T-Tapp.

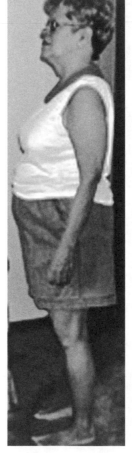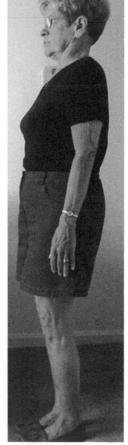

I have also changed the way I eat, adding more whole grains, salads, fresh fruit, etc. The weight has fallen off, especially above my waist, which is where I had trouble losing before. And I couldn't believe it when I went from a 36DD bra to a 34C. Soon I was getting into clothes that I hadn't been able to wear for a very long time.

My husband, who has never had a weight problem, is so proud of me for sticking with this and accomplishing my goals. My "fat" clothes are now in paper bags! It's so nice to look in the mirror and see a normal-sized body. Did I also mention how much fun it is to shop for clothes again?

Although the T-Tapp stance may feel strange at first, it will come to feel natural because this alignment *is* natural. It is also a very safe position. It strengthens and protects your back by providing a solid foundation from which to work. In fact, the reasons this stance feels awkward, at least initially, is because most of us are so out of alignment—we have developed muscle imbalances over time. As a result, we have to retrain our muscles not only to hold the body in better alignment but also to work in synch with full fiber activation.

In terms of inch loss, it's easy to see how this stance can be so effective. Think about how many muscles are engaged. You have isometric contractions everywhere—in the legs and butt, as well as in the upper and lower abs—and you haven't even started to work out!

FOCUS ON FORM

Once you start T-Tapping, remember that it's better to do fewer repetitions with proper form than it is to do more repetitions with poor form. Many newcomers have the impression that if they don't do all the repetitions I recommend, they won't get results. This is not true! We all have our own personal max—depending on fitness level and flexibility—and it's important to push ourselves to that point to get the best results. So if you can manage only four or five repetitions when I recommend eight, that's fine. As long as you go to *your* max and have proper form, you *will* receive rapid results and get stronger. And as you become stronger, you will be able to add more repetitions with good form.

Keep in mind that T-Tapp is a learning process in the beginning, and it's more comprehensive than it looks. But trust me—the more effort you put into proper form, the better results you'll see, both in terms of inch loss and overall health and well-being.

I also want you to understand that T-Tapp is progressive. I don't want you to freak out if your form isn't perfect when you first start to do T-Tapp. Initially, you may not be strong or flexible enough to replicate the exact form as shown in the pictures in this book. Even after you've been T-Tapping for a while, you may have days when you're stronger and more flexible than others, due to lack of sleep, too much stress, not eating well—whatever. The important thing is to do the best you can and recognize that the more you T-Tapp, the more you'll get out of it and the better your form will be. That's the beauty of this workout. As long as you commit to going to *your* personal max every time you do T-Tapp, you will *always* be challenged.

ALWAYS EXERCISE IN SEQUENCE

With most traditional workouts, it doesn't matter which exercise you do first or last, as long as you warm up with some stretching moves. But with T-Tapp, it's important to do the exercises in sequence. Why? First, I've designed these movements to fatigue your muscles layer by layer. So if you don't do them in order, you won't be maximizing your muscles as efficiently as possible, and your results may not be as dramatic. For example, I have you do lunges before balance moves, because I want to fatigue your large leg muscles so that your body is forced to use your deeper, core muscles to maintain balance.

Another reason sequence is important is that the body always uses the path of least resistance, and most of us have stronger leg muscles than core muscles. Taking this concept a step further, fatiguing strong muscles forces you to use weaker muscles so that your body develops all-over muscle strength as well as flexibility.

The sequencing of T-Tapp exercises also allows the body to achieve target heart rate for optimal fat burning along with elimination of excess lactic acid. As a result, your body optimizes Krebs cycle function. In simple terms, the Krebs cycle is a set of enzyme reactions that occur in the body at the cellular level and produce the bulk of your muscles' energy needs. For more detailed information about the Krebs cycle, I recommend reading *Smart Exercise,* by Covert Bailey, Ph.D. Dr. Bailey was my role model when I was in college, and he does an excellent job of simplifying a somewhat complicated subject.

There's one exception to the sequence rule: two T-Tapp exercises, Primary Back Stretch and Hoe Downs, can be done anytime without doing anything else. You'll learn about both of these in the next chapter.

WORK WITH YOUR BODY TYPE

Ever notice how some of us tend to gain weight in our lower bodies, while others tend to carry all of our extra weight in our tummies? We've all heard about "apples" and "pears," but when it comes to anatomical structure, there are more factors involved than just fat deposits that alter our silhouettes to resemble fruit.

While it's true that different body types have different areas where fat tends to accumulate, the good news is that I created T-Tapp to work for *all* body types. Understanding what your body type is can help you know what to focus on while doing each of the T-Tapp exercises so that they will best target *your* areas of concern.

Kiona W. Leah

"T-Tapp has revolutionized my life!"

I hated my hips, my thighs, my flabby, fat stomach! I spent hours agonizing over the bulges on my body. What's sad is that, at the time, I was a comfortable size eight.

I started working out two to three hours a day, six days a week. I followed a strict bodybuilding diet that allowed me a day off every ten days, during which I binged and took harsh laxatives, then did extra cardio the next few days as penance. The thought of putting on even a single ounce terrified me because my self-esteem was tied to my size and shape.

My food binges became more frequent, and I soon ballooned to a size sixteen or even eighteen. In addition to the emotional struggle, I was also beginning to fight a physical one as my liver, kidneys, spleen, pancreas, adrenal glands, and digestive organs all began to function poorly from lack of proper nutrition and crushing stress. Desperate and terrified of who I was and the lie I was living, I found T-Tapp.

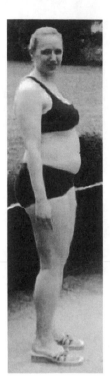

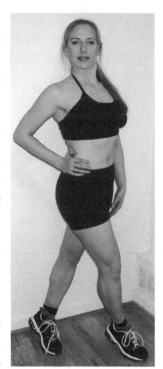

Currently I am a size eight. I now know that my body type will not have slim hips, but I can love and appreciate the natural curves I'm blessed with. My stomach is taut, my saddlebags have been sculpted away, and my voluptuous hips sit atop long, thin legs. My arms have more tone and muscle than they did when I was lifting weights. I enjoy all the foods I want, when I want, and no longer fear gaining weight or losing control. Probably the most profound change for me is that things do not *have to be perfect—like my workout schedule, eating, etc.—and I can still feel good and get great* results.

I've classified body types (or anatomical structures) into three main categories: Short Torso/Long Leg (sometimes referred to as the "apple"), Long Torso/Short Leg (sometimes referred to as the "pear"), and Combination (which can have variations that lean toward either of the previously mentioned body types). Body type has nothing to do with your height. I've met a lot of short people who think they can't possibly be a Long Torso and a lot of tall people who think they can't possibly be a Short Torso. So don't assume that you already know which body type you are. Grab a tape measure, follow the instructions, and find out for sure.

To determine your body type, assume the T-Tapp stance and jot down these dimensions:

1. **Rib to hip:** Measure from the bottom of your very bottom rib (on the side of your body) to the very top of your hipbone. 4"
2. **Knee to ankle:** Measure from your ankle bone, up the side of your leg, to your knee joint. 14"
3. **Knee to hip:** Measure the distance from your knee joint to your hip joint. *Note:* Finding your top measuring point on this one can be a bit tricky. I recommend standing up and doing a side 14"

leg lift. The point where your leg lifts on the side of your body is your top measuring point. Going down the side of your body, measure from that point to your knee.

Now let's see where you fall.

You're a Long Torso/Short Leg Body Type If . . .

- The distance from your rib to hip measures six to eight inches or greater.
- The distance from your knee to ankle is *less* than the distance from your knee to hip.
- You tend to gain weight on the outer thighs and butt.

A longer torso allows for plenty of room for internal organs, so it's easier to maintain a flat stomach and for the obliques to cinch in and

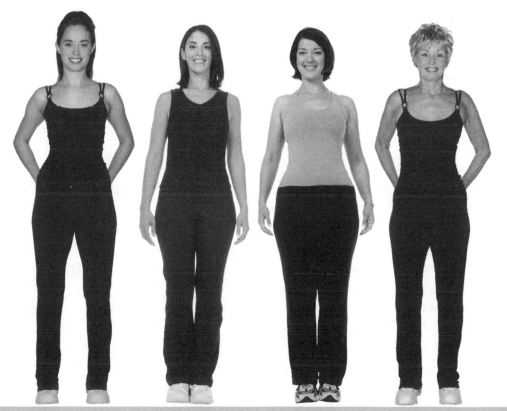

create a slim waistline. Additionally, a Long Torso's derriere shape tends to "bubble" and be more round instead of flat. But this body type commonly battles cellulite, even when fit.

Long Torso/Short Leg body types have a high tendency to become disproportionate—inchwise, the lower body is usually bigger than the upper body. This is my body type, so I know from experience that we Long Torsos tend to carry one or two inches more in our hips than we do in our bust. In high school, I used to wear a size six top and a size ten or twelve bottom, and I was an in-shape cheerleader and soccer player! Today, thanks to T-Tapp, I wear a size four or six, top *and* bottom. But for many Long Torso/Short Leg body types, a difference of one or two inches between the bust and hip is not unusual, even after T-Tapping.

However, if this body type gets out of shape, it can almost look like they have two different bodies put together. Fortunately, T-Tapp can make a dramatic difference.

You're a Short Torso/Long Leg Body Type If . . .

- The distance from your rib to hip measures two inches or less.
- The distance from your knee to ankle is equal to or greater than the distance from your knee to hip.
- You tend to gain weight along the inner thighs and lower tummy.

A Short Torso's backside tends to be more flat than round, and this body type doesn't get saddlebags or carry extra weight in the hips and thighs. Short Torsos are the ones you will hear referred to as having "legs up to their eyeballs." Cellulite is usually not a big problem for Short Torso/Long Leg body types, but since distance from the hips to the ribs is shorter, that means less room is available for internal organs. As a result, waistlines are typically thicker, and tummies tend to bulge. Even models with short torsos worry about lower tummy pooch. Add childbirth to the equation, and not only does the lower abdominal cavity expand, but so does the rib cage. And when there's only an inch or so between the ribs and hip, a barrel chest can occur.

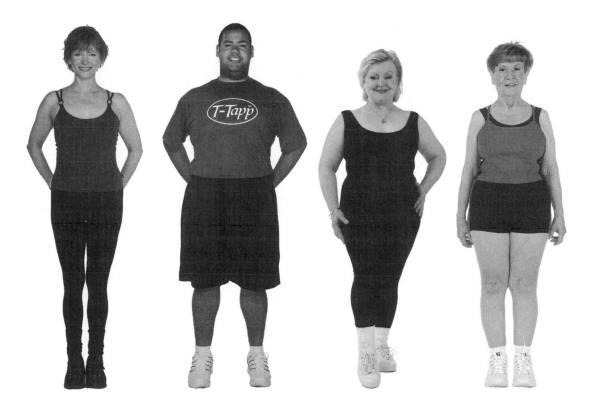

Less distance from the ribs to the hips tends to cause a Short Torso to arch the butt as well—like a gymnast does at the end of a routine—to make more room for the belly. However, arching the butt inactivates muscles at the top of the hip, which creates a tendency to store fat there (commonly referred to as "hip pads"). Arching the butt also causes the abdominal organs to push forward and down, thus creating lower tummy pooch. And just like the Long Torso/Short Leg, this body type can also be disproportionate—except in this case, the upper body is typically one to two inches larger than the lower body.

The Short Torso's longer knee-to-ankle distance makes this person more susceptible to a condition called pronation of the knees, where the feet aim outward but the knees roll inward. As a result, Short Torsos may often stand and walk knock-kneed. Unfortunately, when the knees roll inward, so do the hips, and muscular imbalance begins.

Therefore, fat storage occurs at the inside of the knee (often called "knee-knocker fat"), and the knees may start to hurt.

You're a Combination Body Type If . . .

- The distance from your rib to hip measures five inches.
- The distance from your knee to ankle is equal to the distance from your knee to hip.
- You tend to gain weight in the butt and gut, as well as the inner thigh. You're also prone to back fat and hip pads (lower back area above the butt), as well as what's known as a "third butt cheek," meaning there's often a small "bun" just below the butt cheek.

Extra pounds tend to be more evenly distributed on Combos, and it's fairly easy for this body type to maintain overall proportions. However, there's a tendency for Combos to have a small roll of fat below the belly button and to carry more meat on their upper arms.

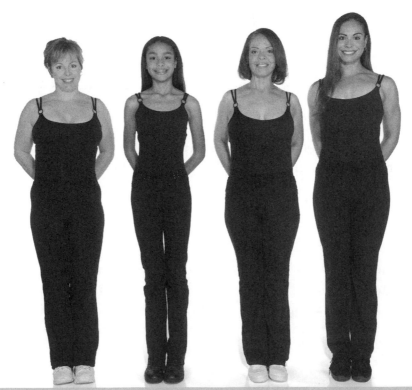

There are variations within the Combination body type in that Combos can lean toward being a Short or Long Torso. To determine if you're one of those varieties, keep reading.

If the distance from your rib to hip is closer to five and one-half or six inches and the distance from your knee to ankle is less than the distance of your knee to hip, you would be classified as a Combo with Long Torso tendencies. If the distance from your rib to hip is closer than three inches and your knee to ankle distance is equal to or greater than the distance from your knee to hip, you would be classified as a Combo with Short Torso tendencies. Overall, it's important to think of these body types as guidelines rather than rigid categories, because you may very well fall somewhere in between.

So, why does body type matter? In the modeling world, it matters—especially in terms of swimsuits. Long Torsos always wear bikinis well but never high-cut, one-piece suits, whereas Short Torsos always look fantastic in high-cut swimsuits, but not so good in bikinis. True Combos can wear any style swimsuit and look fabulous, but a Combo

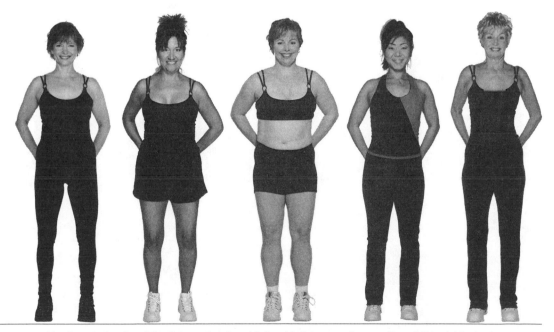

Here's a photo of each body type standing side by side for easy reference. From left to right: short torso, combo bordering on short torso, true combo, combo bordering on long torso, long torso

with a Short Torso will look cuter in a high-waisted two-piece, and a Combo Long Torso will look great in a string bikini, but not as great in a two-piece suit with boy-cut legs.

For the rest of us, body type matters mostly in terms of realistic expectations. If you're a Long Torso, for example, you'll likely always have trouble with saddlebags, but you can also achieve a waistline to die for. If you're a Short Torso, you may never have a tiny waist, no matter how many oblique exercises you do, but you're likely to always have great-looking legs, even as you age. And as a Combo, it's easier for you to hide weight gain, so you're always going to look good in clothes.

What's important here is to set your sights on a goal that will put your *own* body into proportion rather than worrying about getting your waist size down to that of a model or a friend you might admire (okay, *envy* may be a better word) but whose body type may be completely different from yours.

The bottom line is that we all have something about our bodies we may not love that will always be with us, but it's part of who we are. For me, no matter how fit I am, I'm always challenged with outer thigh

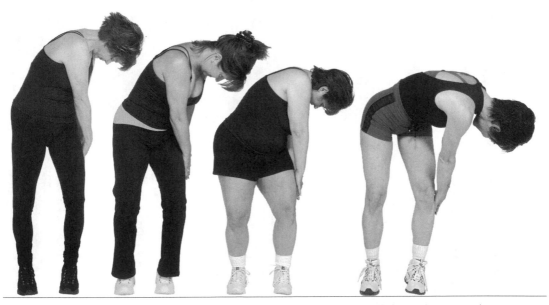

Left to right: short torso, combo bordering on short torso, combo bordering on long torso, long torso

bulge—known as the stubborn saddlebags. But at least T-Tapp helps me keep these under control. In fact, the terrific thing about T-Tapp is that no matter what your body type is, you'll end up with a body that is sculpted and more proportionate. It's all about muscle mechanics, no matter how long or how short your bones are.

It's important for you to be educated about body types, not only because it helps you to set realistic, achievable goals for yourself, but also because your range of motion within some T-Tapp movements may differ, depending on which body type you are. In the T-Tapp Twist, for example, a Long Torso may be able to reach past the knee, but even on a good day, a Short Torso may not be able to get past midthigh without losing butt tuck. Or, with Thread the Needle, Short Torsos may not be able to get their legs over as far as a Long Torso can, because there's simply not as much space from rib to hips. So do take the time to figure out which body type you are so that you can achieve maximum benefits from each exercise.

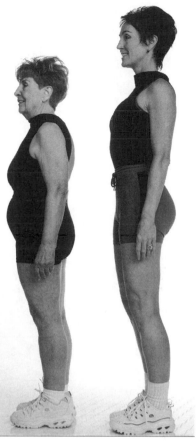

Notice how the distance from the knee to the ankle is the same even though we are different heights and different body types.

Lisa Wallace

"T-Tapp made shopping fun again!"

I am so excited, and I have to share! I started seriously T-Tapping at the beginning of this year (January 4, to be exact). With the exception of a few weeks of illness during this time, I was very consistent about working out. In just twelve

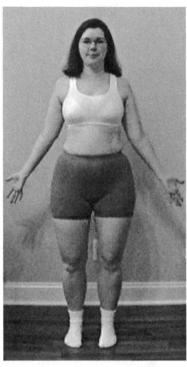
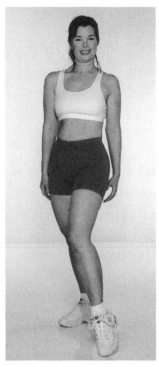

weeks, my size twelve or fourteen pants were literally hanging off me, so I decided to treat myself to some new ones.

I took a size ten and a size eight to the dressing room. I tried on the size ten first. Way too big! Grinning from ear to ear, I tried on the size eight. Also too big! In shock, I returned those pants to the rack and took a size six and a size four into the dressing room. The size six pair fit perfectly. I could not believe it! Just for fun, I tried the size four pair on. I was able to get them up and zipped, and I was able to bend, squat, and sit in them with no problem (all of this while still breathing)! But they were really too tight for wearing out in public at my age. I did buy a pair of the size four for inspiration, though. I am just so thrilled that I am back in a size six. I haven't been below a size ten since I became pregnant with my first child!

To anyone who is questioning if T-Tapp really works, the answer is a resounding yes! *It absolutely does work, and I have new pants to prove it!*

TAKE YOUR MEASUREMENTS

Before starting to T-Tapp, it's important for you to measure yourself. That way, you can track your progress as you lose inches and feel motivated to continue working out. I recommend remeasuring yourself once a week and keeping a record of your workout schedule as well.

For accurate measurements, assume the T-Tapp stance and tighten your muscles while measuring. Stand with your feet spaced directly under your hip joints with toes forward and knees slightly bent and pushing out toward the little toe. Keep your butt tucked with shoulders back and in alignment with hip joints at all times, except when measuring lower thighs and calves.

Here's where to measure:

- **Bust:** fullest part of bust
- **Pecs:** just above the bust line
- **Ribs:** top of rib cage just below the bust line
- **Waist:** at or slightly above the navel

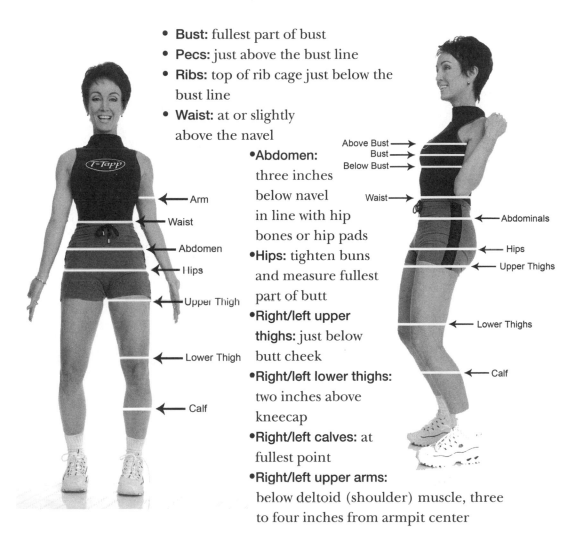

- •**Abdomen:** three inches below navel in line with hip bones or hip pads
- •**Hips:** tighten buns and measure fullest part of butt
- •**Right/left upper thighs:** just below butt cheek
- •**Right/left lower thighs:** two inches above kneecap
- •**Right/left calves:** at fullest point
- •**Right/left upper arms:** below deltoid (shoulder) muscle, three to four inches from armpit center

YOUR PERSONAL MEASURING CHART

	STARTING MEASUREMENTS	WEEK ONE	WEEK TWO	WEEK THREE	WEEK FOUR
BUST: fullest part of bust	42		41¾		
PECS: just above the bust line	41		39.5		
RIBS: top of rib cage just below the bust line	36.5		36		
WAIST: at or slightly above the navel	41		41		
ABDOMEN: three inches below the navel in line with hip bones or hip pads	45.5		45.5		
HIPS: tighten buns and measure fullest part of butt	45.5		47.5		
UPPER THIGHS: just below butt cheek R	25½		25		
L	24		24		
LOWER THIGHS: two inches above knee cap R	18		18		
L	17.5		18		
CALVES: at fullest point R	14.5		15		
L	14.75		14.5		
UPPER ARMS: below deltoid (shoulder) muscle, three to four inches from armpit center R	13		14		
L	12.5		13		

GET READY FOR BOOT CAMP

With T-Tapp, you can lose inches quickly by doing nothing more than my fifteen-minute Basic Plus Workout three days a week. But if you want to kickstart your inch loss or have a specific goal you need to achieve by a certain date, I recommend you start the T-Tapp program with a four-to-fourteen-day boot camp. That means working out every day for as long as your chosen boot camp lasts. The length of your boot camp depends on how many clothing sizes you would like to lose.

To tighten and tone and/or lose one clothing size:
- Do a full T-Tapp workout (fifteen-minute Basic Plus Workout or forty-five minute Total Workout) four days in a row.
- Then switch to an every-other-day workout schedule for two to three weeks.
- Then take two days off between workouts for two to three weeks.
- Once you have reached your desired clothing size, work out once or twice a week to maintain results.

To lose two clothing sizes:
- Do a full T-Tapp workout (fifteen-minute Basic Plus Workout or forty-five minute Total Workout) seven days in a row.
- Then switch to an every-other-day workout schedule for two to three weeks.
- Then take two days off between workouts for another three to four weeks.
- Once you have reached your desired clothing size, work out once or twice a week to maintain results.

To lose three clothing sizes:
- Do a full T-Tapp workout (fifteen-minute Basic Plus Workout or forty-five-minute Total Workout) ten days in a row.
- Then switch to an every-other-day workout schedule for four to five weeks.

- Then take two days off between workouts for another four to five weeks. Once you have reached your desired clothing size, work out once or twice a week to maintain results.

To lose four or more clothing sizes:

- Do a full T-Tapp workout (fifteen-minute Basic Plus Workout or forty-five minute Total Workout) fourteen days in a row.
- Then switch to an every-other-day workout schedule for four to five weeks.
- Then take two days off between workouts for another four to five weeks.
- Once you have reached your desired clothing size, work out once or twice a week to maintain results.

For optimal results during boot camp, focus on just doing T-Tapp exercises. Walking as little or as much as you'd like is fine, but avoid doing any other workouts, such as weight lifting, aerobics, Pilates, and so on. I'm going to be teaching you new techniques to maximize muscle movement, and your body will respond better without interference from other exercises.

During boot camp, your body is literally rebuilding neurokinetic connections throughout your muscles, layer by layer, from the inside out. Boot camp also forces your body to use muscles you rarely use in daily activity, which is why we atrophy from the inside out as we age.

During boot camp, there's a significant exchange of fat for muscle, and although it varies from person to person, in my twenty-five years of teaching T-Tapp, I've noticed statistical patterns. The average person will gain five to seven pounds of muscle within one week, and at the same time lose seven to ten pounds of body fat. This exchange may not show on a scale, but it will be revealed in inch loss. That five to seven pounds of muscle is intrinsic muscle core—and that's what will stoke that new fat-burning furnace at an average of 250 to 350 calories more per day without any change in diet. But you must T-Tapp at least four days in a row to get that internal core density.

Melissa Poe

"I dropped two sizes in two weeks!"

As a former fashion model, I have always been thin and never really had to watch what I ate. All that changed when I turned thirty-two, gained fourteen pounds in three months, and went from a size six to a ten. I blamed it on my doctor changing my birth control pills. I started working out harder, which meant adding more cardio to my routine for four days a week. After six weeks with no results, I increased that to six or seven days a week. After three more months and no results at all, I was beginning to believe I was never going to lose the weight and that I would have to start dieting. Over the next year, I bought every weight-loss pill on the market and tried different exercise programs, to no avail. It was extremely depressing to know that if I wanted to model again, I couldn't because of my weight gain.

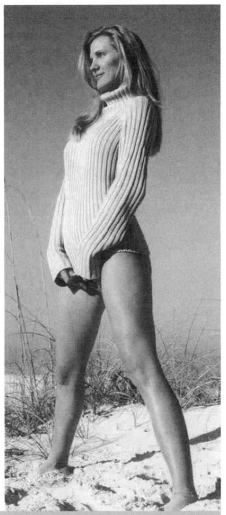

I started searching the Internet for some kind of wellness program—if I couldn't look good, then maybe I could feel good. My search results took me to the T-Tapp Web site. Everything I read sounded too good to be true, but the T-Tapp name rang a bell. I soon realized I'd overheard other models talking about this workout, so I decided to give it a try.

After doing just a few moves from the fifteen-minute workout for ten days, I lost an inch off each upper thigh and an inch off my abdomen. You can imagine my excitement! Results were even more dramatic after two weeks of doing the Total Workout: I dropped two clothing sizes and was back into a size six.

On days one and two of boot camp, take things slowly, and really focus on proper form. By day three, you might be calling me names—that's why T-Tapp is an at-home fitness program! But by day four, the exercises will be much easier. That's because your body will break through a physiological plateau—which is the very reason why it's so important to do the workout at least four days in a row at the beginning, or after going six weeks or more without T-Tapping. Boot camps are also a great way to supercharge your workout or break through inch-loss plateaus.

Note: You may feel slightly nauseated the first time you do the workout. This is because T-Tapp is *so* lymphatic, and your body is ridding itself of stored toxins. Drinking water or eating an apple will usually help when you feel this way. But do not sit or lie down, as that could make you feel worse. Instead, walk it out.

One of the amazing benefits of T-Tapp is that once you rebuild that neurokinetic connection and some of that internal density, it's easy to maintain. That's why you do a boot camp—to rebuild. Then you can get great results by working out every other day before going to every third day as you get closer to your goal. T-Tapp is like a reward system. In the beginning, you're rebuilding and turning back time. Then, once you've rebuilt your body to work more efficiently, it's easier to maintain, and ultimately you'll only have to work out twice a week (depending on what you eat) to stay trim and feel terrific.

Will you be sore after you do T-Tapp? Most likely. I've heard many die-hard fitness fanatics claim they're not worried about getting sore from my workout because they're in such good shape. But most *do* get sore, because their bodies are not accustomed to using T-Tapp techniques. The best remedy for soreness? I recommend treating yourself to a warm bath with Dead Sea salts. Salt soaks are also great for your skin, so it's a win-win, inside and out.

REMEMBER TO BREATHE!

Proper breathing (inhaling through the nose, exhaling through the mouth) is particularly important when you T-Tapp. More oxygen in your bloodstream gives you more energy as well as a (much welcome) chance to pause and refocus on form and the exercise you're performing. Most of us habitually get only a third of the oxygen that we're capable of taking in. Yet oxygen triggers countless chemical reactions in the body that can help you get trim and feel terrific. For instance, when oxygen reaches fat molecules, it breaks them down into carbon dioxide and water. The carbon dioxide is then exhaled, the water flushed away, and the fat is gone for good!

Deep breathing also helps your lymphatic system work more efficiently. The toxins collected throughout the body drain through two ducts situated at the base of the neck and the thoracic duct. Breathing drives this action. In other words, by taking deep breaths, you're massaging the thoracic duct upward into the neck so that fluid flows generously. This duct empties the lymph into the veins, where it becomes part of the blood plasma. From there, the lymph returns to the liver for metabolization, and finally to the kidneys for filtering.

Sherry Richard

She blew away an extra two inches!

My body type is Short Torso/Long Leg, so I've always battled lower belly bulge and a barrel chest. After I delivered twins, my rib cage really expanded. When I started T-Tapping, I measured thirty-eight inches around my bra line.

T-Tapp helped me to lose two inches, but then I plateaued. That's when I started really focusing on deep breathing while T-Tapping. Once I got the hang

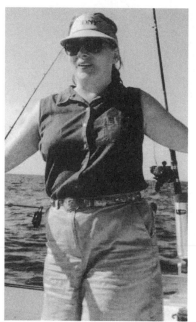

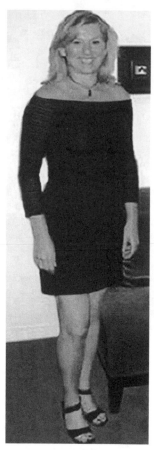

*of fully expanding my rib cage while inhaling and fully contracting it while exhaling, I lost an ad*ditional *two inches. It took about two months, but I've always been a slow loser.*

During many of the exercises in this book, I'm going to tell you to "inhale big, exhale bigger"—and here's why. As you age, atrophy tends to occur in the muscles between the ribs, often due to shallow breathing, which causes the rib cage to expand. This is why so many men and women get thicker waistlines and barrel chests as they get older. However, women who have had children suffer even more, because while the fetus is growing, it not only stretches the uterus, it expands the rib cage as well—especially in women with shorter torsos.

When you inhale big (until you feel your ribs stretch) and exhale bigger (all the way until your lungs empty the oxygen and you pull your ribs together), you're getting full extension and full contraction of the muscles between the ribs. This enables you to completely stretch the muscle fibers and build muscle density. In fact, since this deep breathing technique compresses muscles between your ribs, it's an exercise in itself, because when you tighten and tone these torso muscles, they cinch in like a corset.

The best way to check your breathing is to practice first in front of a mirror. Inhale slowly while focusing on expanding the diaphragm area above the belly button. Make an effort to expand the sides of the body as well. Then exhale slowly, as if you were blowing through a straw, and try to compress the rib bones together in the middle. Your objective here is to pull the sides together as much as possible in and down the torso. Always exhale for at least twice as long as you inhale, and really pull, pull, pull the ribs together.

When you expand your sides during an inhale and compress them during an exhale, this gives your abdominal muscles as well as the muscles between the ribs a wonderful workout. In fact, if you stick with this kind of breathing whenever you T-Tapp, you'll likely see an inch or more disappear off your rib cage within seven to ten days!

DRINK PLENTY OF WATER BEFORE, DURING, AND AFTER T-TAPPING

Water is important for hydration, of course, but it also does wonders for your waistline. When you drink water, it goes to the stomach, then filters out into the internal network throughout the body—including the lymphatic system. From there, it not only washes the cells, organs, and kidneys, but also helps to move things out—including excess liquefied fat that is being transported throughout your body. It also flushes out toxic waste in your system and keeps your body functioning efficiently.

REAL PEOPLE, REAL RESULTS

Margit Mehne

With T-Tapp, you don't have to be a fitness fanatic!

I've always enjoyed exercise and found it fairly easy to stay in shape with walking, yoga, and aerobics. But once I turned thirty, the pounds and cellulite began to accumulate. I followed a serious strength-training workout, which only made me look worse—causing me to trade in size eight jeans for fourteen. I spent the next several years trying unsuccessfully to reverse the bulk with a variety of workouts and diets. When my weight peaked at around 180, I turned to light weights and aerobics, which I faithfully followed for two years. That gave me limited re-

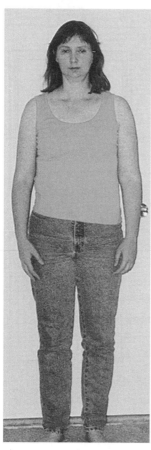
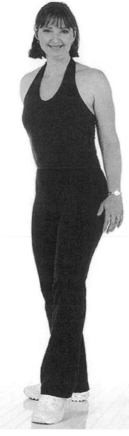

sults as long as I exercised very strenuously almost daily. My weight came down, but I still looked dumpy, was often sick, felt hungry all the time, and was in a perpetual bad mood.

After just one month of T-Tapp, however, the cellulite from my arms disappeared completely, and the rest was beginning to diminish. The workouts were intense, yet they left me feeling exhilarated rather than drained. Once I began to understand that I was rebuilding body systems and muscles from the inside, it became even more motivating. I've always made the effort to exercise, but this unique workout went deeper than others, working with my body rather than against it.

The changes I'd been hoping for followed. I slimmed down and tightened up. I have lost sixteen and a half inches from my midsection to the upper thighs and now wear a size ten. Best of all, at forty, I'm finally able to live a more balanced life—with time for other *interests besides fitness!*

When you don't drink enough water, your kidneys can't function properly, so your liver is forced to help the kidneys out. This diverts the liver from its primary duty, which is transforming fat into fuel. Thus your fat loss stops, or at the very least plateaus.

Drinking water has been shown to boost your metabolism as well. Recent studies at the University of Utah, for example, reveal that even mild dehydration (drinking four eight-ounce glasses of water or less per day) can cause the body's calorie-burning powers to plummet by as much as 2 percent. However, subjects who drank eight or twelve glasses of water a day not only reported better concentration and more energy, they also burned more calories at rest than those who drank only four glasses.

In another study, conducted at the Volhard Clinical Research Center in Berlin, Germany, scientists found that after subjects drank seventeen ounces of water, their metabolic rate increased by 30 percent within ten minutes—and didn't peak until about forty minutes later.

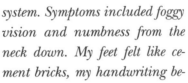

REAL PEOPLE, REAL RESULTS

Heather Petrie

"I found relief for my MS!"

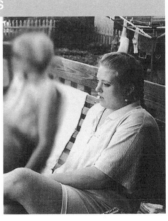

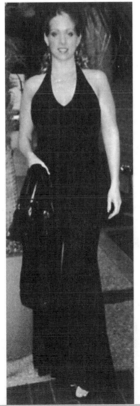

Five years ago, I had my first onset of multiple sclerosis (MS), an autoimmune disease that attacks the nervous system. Symptoms included foggy vision and numbness from the neck down. My feet felt like cement bricks, my handwriting became large and loopy, and I had the sensation that my diaphragm was being squeezed. I was stuttering and slurring a bit and had short-term memory loss. I was dropping everything because I couldn't sense how tightly I was gripping, or my hand would just let the object go. At night, I would have light flashes when I closed my eyes, and my head jerked.

I visited three doctors and kept getting unacceptable responses to my symptoms—everything from telling me to come back in a month if I didn't feel better to taking an aspirin. I had recently lost over 115 pounds, but the weight had started to creep back on, despite the fact that I was running two miles twice a day, lifting weights an hour a day, doing the elliptical trainer for thirty minutes, and drinking protein drinks as meal replacements. I was starving, not seeing the results I wanted—and wow, did the MS flare up! But I was desperate not to gain the weight back.

When I found T-Tapp, I was wearing a size twelve and was mostly concerned with losing weight. Not only did that happen (I'm now wearing a size eight), but my MS improved! And no wonder! What could be better for a person with a neurological disorder than to get the neurokinetic flow going and pumping the lymphatic system?

Drinking water may help to curb your appetite as well. Oftentimes when you get a hunger pang, you're actually feeling dehydrated. So the next time you feel hungry between meals, try drinking a glass of water and see if your hunger goes away.

ABOVE ALL, REMEMBER THAT INCHES COUNT, POUNDS DON'T!

I know I sound like a broken record, but I want to make sure you get this message loud and clear. I don't want you to fret if the scale hasn't budged—or even if it's gone up—after you've been T-Tapping for two weeks or more. Instead, I want you to focus on how much looser your clothes feel and how much more energy you have. With T-Tapp, it's very common to lose a dozen or so inches without any weight loss.

REAL PEOPLE, REAL RESULTS

Diane Stone

"I'm a T-Tapper for life!"

I'm in my mid-forties, and for the first time since puberty, I have maintained the same weight and size for over three years. Thanks to T-Tapp, my entire life has improved in ways that I never dreamed possible.

I was a very active child and teenager who rode horses every day and com-

peted in horse shows regularly. When I stopped riding, my ongoing fight to lose weight became a serious issue in my life.

In 1982, I participated in a residential diet program in Durham, North Carolina, and lost eighty pounds in five months by following an 800-calorie-per-

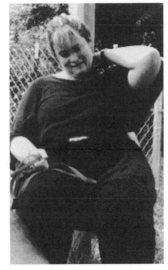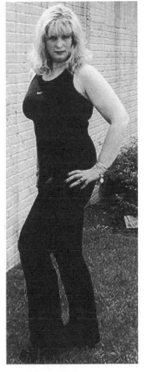

day diet and walking up to twenty miles per day. I was super-thin and super-fit aerobically, but my muscle tone and flexibility left a lot to be desired.

I eventually gained back all of that weight plus more. By January 2000, I was finally ready to get back in shape. At the time, I was wearing a size thirty women's. I began my fitness quest by following a cardio and weight training regimen and lost several sizes before starting T-Tapp.

But T-Tapp has shaped my body like no other exercise program ever could. I no longer live by the numbers on the scale, and because I have so much long, lean muscle, my weight bears little relation to my size. The last time I wore the size I wear now—a twelve or fourteen tall—I was thirty pounds lighter! My body is better proportioned, stronger, and more flexible than at any time in the past. Best of all, I'm back jumping horses and loving every minute of it.

Keep in mind that muscle weighs more than the same volume of fat would, so initially you're going to *look* like you've lost a lot more weight than what the scale says. That's because those tight, dense muscles you've been building take up less space than bulky muscle or fatty flab would. And since those newfound muscles also burn fat for fuel, eventually weight loss *does* occur.

In terms of looking fit and feeling fabulous, dramatic inch loss is always preferable to dramatic weight loss. Dramatic weight loss can leave you feeling weak, tired, and more prone to health problems, while dramatic inch loss—through the loss of fat and the increase of tight, dense muscle mass—leaves you feeling healthier, more fit, and ready to enjoy life to the fullest.

Perhaps Lannette Madden sums it up best when she poses this question: "If you could shed 100 pounds, but that drop in weight would only result in a loss of three inches, or you could choose to lose sixty inches, but the scale would reflect only a five-pound weight loss, which would you choose?"

If you ask me, *that's* a no-brainer!

LOG ON!

Every exercise in this book is accompanied by detailed instructions and illustrations. However, I've also provided a proof-of-purchase coupon on the last page of this book that you can mail in to receive information that will enable you to visit my Web site (www.t-tapp.com) and obtain free technical support by telephone or e-mail, along with the ability to purchase T-Tapp workouts at a 30% discount. At the Web site, which is pop-up-free, you'll also find hundreds of informative articles, as well as free forums where T-Tappers compare progress and encourage one another. Unlike most interactive sites, your comments appear right away, so you can chat live—and make friends—with T-Tappers from all over the world!

REAL PEOPLE, REAL RESULTS

Judy Read

"Now men are whistling at me!"

I recently gained an extra twenty pounds on top of the weight I had been carrying around for the last two years. The stress of a divorce and coping with a house that needed so many repairs really got to me, and I just ate and ate and ate. For

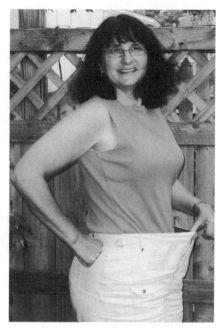

the first time in my life, I got a stomach roll and felt like I was carrying around a Jell-O factory! None of my nice clothes fit anymore, so I rotated through the same four makeshift outfits for work.

When I went for my yearly cardiology checkup, the doctor said he would give me a year to take the weight off, then we would "talk." I have a prolapsed valve, and the uphills are tough enough for me without carrying around a permanent built-in weight pack. My mother is a type 2 diabetic, and that black cloud has been hanging over my head as well.

I decided to start T-Tapping with a fourteenday boot camp of Basic Plus Workout. By the end, my stomach had shrunk dramatically. Soon I was wearing shorts and a tank top and started to feel really good about myself. Over the next six weeks, I lost eighteen inches—a whole shorts size—and when I recently visited New Mexico, men whistled at me!

I love Primary Back Stretch! It has really improved my posture. When I drive, I use that time to work my shoulders and lats. It's a huge fatigue fighter. T-Tapp has given me a more upbeat outlook on life. I'm happier and more content, and I feel like I can accomplish things!

Elliott Martin

"I found my lats!"

When I first started T-Tapping, I did the Basic Plus Workout five out of seven days the first week. Right away, I noticed I was feeling better. I had more energy and was sleeping better. Then I sliced up the bottom of my foot—no KLT!

It took me over three weeks to heal, after which I got back to my T-Tapp routine. I didn't change my eating habits at all. After working out for four weeks, I had lost six and a half inches total and gained a half inch in each arm—which for a man is a good thing. I noticed other improvements as well: better posture, more defined shoulders and deltoids (I found my lats!), and more flexibility, along with the increased energy. I also found that the workouts got harder each time when I focused on keeping the tuck and my shoulders back. I plan to stick with this routine so that I can be in even better shape by the end of the year!

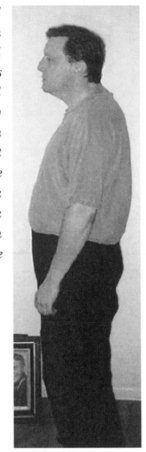
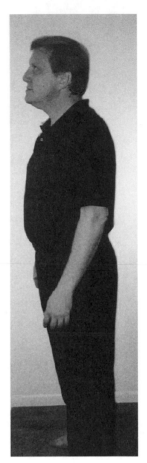

4

The T-Tapp
Basic Plus Workout

T-Tapp's Basic Plus Workout is designed primarily for beginners and
to help the fit get fitter. It delivers inch loss as well as improved
health and wellness. This quickie workout tightens and tones, strengthens and stretches, de-stresses and energizes—plus saves time. It takes
just fifteen minutes to complete, yet still provides cardiac conditioning
and improved circulation.

There's an interesting story behind this time-saving routine.
Based on my formal education, all the research I had read, and my own
personal experiences, I used to believe that you had to exercise for at
least forty-five minutes to burn fat and lose inches. Then three years
ago, WMAR-TV, an ABC affiliate in Baltimore, Maryland, invited view-
ers to enter a drawing for a fitness challenge. The winner would receive
a videotape of my forty-five-minute Total Workout, and the television

station would report on his or her results after thirty days. A fifty-two-year-old woman was declared the winner, and right away—on live TV—she insisted that she didn't have forty-five minutes a day to exercise. However, she did promise to do the first fifteen minutes of my Total Workout for four consecutive days, then switch to an every-other-day routine for the remainder of the month.

Was I worried that she wouldn't see any results? You'd better believe it! Was I surprised when she lost almost two clothing sizes in thirty days? Most definitely! What made these results even sweeter was that this thirty-day challenge occurred during the Christmas holidays—a time when most of us *gain* weight and have no time to exercise.

"I ate cookies and pie and still lost inches," the contest winner declared after the thirty days were up. In fact, she continued to T-Tapp, and within six weeks had lost another size and a half.

These dramatic results made me realize that less really *is* more with T-Tapp. And when testimonials from other T-Tappers with time constraints began pouring in, along with claims that they, too, were getting amazing results from doing just the first fifteen minutes of my Total Workout, I decided to create the Basic Plus Workout.

Enjoy the exercises in this chapter as a stand-alone workout, as a warm-up for my Total Workout (presented in Chapter 5), or on days you're pressed for time but still want to be fit and feel fabulous.

PRIMARY BACK STRETCH

I consider Primary Back Stretch to be one of the most important, if not *the* most important, movement in terms of how much it can help the body help itself build or rebuild neurokinetic and lymphatic function. It can be used as a stand-alone exercise to help your body maintain better spinal alignment with improved strength and flexibility, or it can be used as an effective warm-up to any exercise activity.

Initially, I created Primary Back Stretch to help my body maintain a strong spine with less lower back pain and discomfort, as well as to help cancer patients I was working with to lessen some of the side effects they were experiencing from chemotherapy and radiation treatments. But I discovered over time that when Primary Back Stretch is done before physical activity, it can significantly improve metabolic processing and cardiac performance. Traditional exercise teaches that it takes approximately twenty minutes of activity for the body to warm up, but when you do Primary Back Stretch first, your body turns into a fat-burning machine much quicker.

In addition to contributing to increased endurance and faster fat burning, Primary Back Stretch also offers a multitude of health benefits, such as better circulation with warmer hands and feet, better lymphatic function with less swelling or edema, improved mental clarity with fewer headaches, and improved energy for those with autoimmune disorders. Many people have shared tremendous testimonials on how effective Primary Back Stretch has been for their health. But the amazing part to me isn't the movement—it's the body's ability to respond and repair. That's why it's never too late to get fit or improve your health. However, you must move to make it happen, and when you use comprehensive, compound muscle movement in sequences such as Primary Back Stretch, you enable your body to maximize function and build a better body.

Application of form is very important, so read all the instructions and study the photos before trying this exercise. You should feel heat radiate through your spine and all through your body as you progressively warm up. Best of all, the more neurokinetically connected your body becomes, the faster you will feel this, even to the back of your hands and tops of your feet. Isn't it amazing how three minutes of muscle movement can do so much? I may go days or weeks without doing a full workout, but I always start and finish each day with Primary Back Stretch. See what it can do for you.

Step 1

Assume the T-Tapp stance as explained in Chapter 3, with toes forward, knees bent, butt tucked, shoulders back, and knees out into KLT position. Your hands should be below your waist with fingers lifting away and elbows pulling back as you push your thumbs into your back. Feel how the muscles in your back tightened and how your shoulders pulled back? I call this push/pull action "leverage isometrics" and use it to help your body increase neurokinetic transmission and maximize muscle contraction. Leverage isometrics not only helps establish better isometric activation along the spine and throughout your back, but also

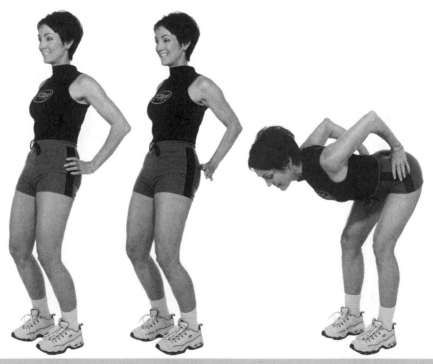

helps create full fiber activation in the muscles from your shoulder to neck (trapezius and latissimus dorsi). Bringing shoulders back in linear alignment to your hips while pushing knees out toward your little toes (KLT) comprehensively activates your abdominal muscles as well. Now arch your butt up as you move your upper body into a flat back position. Keep pushing your thumbs into your back and pull your elbows up. You should feel as though your back is scooped out, 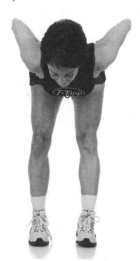 although it appears flat. Inhale/exhale and then tighten your butt. Feel how this intensifies the muscle activation down the back of your thighs? Isometric activation of your gluteal muscles while knees are in KLT optimizes stretch of your hamstring muscles, which in turn burns off more glucose and/or fat. Now inhale bigger and exhale bigger, and proceed to Step 2.

Form Check Shoulders and hips should be level not only for spinal support, but also to maximize effectiveness.

MOST COMMON MISTAKE

If your shoulders are higher or lower than the hips, and if your elbows aren't up, this inactivates your abdominal and back muscles. Linear alignment of shoulder to hip is important.

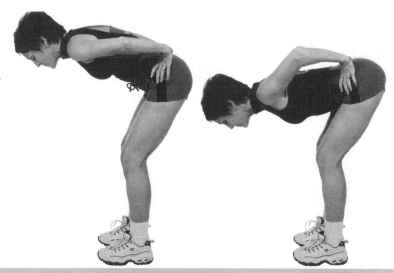

Step 2

While maintaining your upper body in a level position with right knee bent and pushing out to KLT, try to straighten your left leg to the best of your ability with both knees turned out and hold for two counts. Now bend both knees a bit deeper (pushing out in KLT) without losing the flat back position. Inhale as you straighten and exhale as you bend. In-

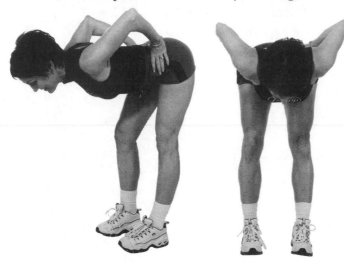

hale again while you straighten your right leg to the best of your ability and exhale as you bend.

Form Check Always keep your hips level and your knees pushing out in KLT position at all times without shifting your weight. Strength and flexibility come with time, so the focus is not so much on getting your leg perfectly straight as it is on straightening your leg to your personal max without allowing either knee to roll in toward the big toe.

MOST COMMON MISTAKES

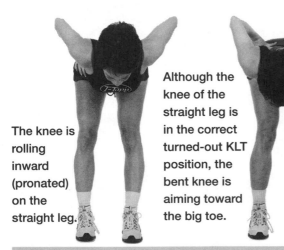

The knee is rolling inward (pronated) on the straight leg.

Although the knee of the straight leg is in the correct turned-out KLT position, the bent knee is aiming toward the big toe.

Although both knees are in the correct position, the shoulders and hips have lost linear alignment. Furthermore, allowing the hip to lift when straightening the leg inactivates the muscles and allows the weight of the body to shift.

Now repeat the entire sequence (left leg then right leg) and proceed to Step 3.

Step 3

Place hands above your knees with thumbs in and fingers out for proper shoulder alignment. You should feel the weight of your upper body pushing into your knees along with a release of muscle tension in your lower back.

MOST COMMON MISTAKE

Fingers in will pronate your shoulder!

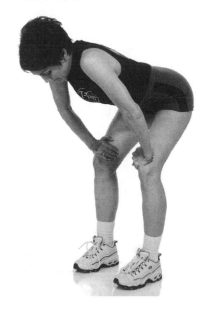

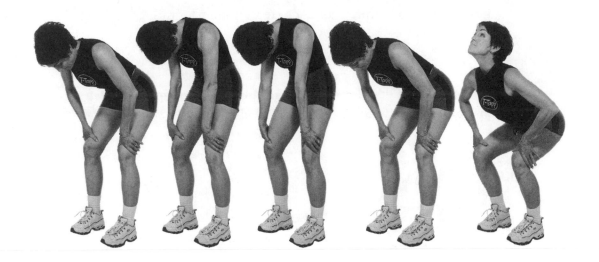

Step 4

Tuck your butt and chin as you push your hands into your knees until your arms straighten, as shown in the first three images. Look closely and compare the elbow and shoulder positions in the second and third images. Once your arms are straight, push your thumbs into your thighs above your knees and twist your elbows in and pull your shoulders back. Inhale big and as you exhale, push your thumbs and pull your shoulders back even more (two counts). Inhale again, but during the exhale scoop your back out and reach your chin up for a reverse spinal stretch (two counts).

Form Check Your body weight should be on your hands, above the knees, to support your spine, and your knees should be pushing out to max KLT. On the exhale, be sure to really reach with your chin.

Repeat Step 4 for a total of two tuck/curl and reach/scoops. Then proceed to Step 5.

Step 5

Repeat tuck/curl sequence once more with another inhale and exhale after you twist your elbows in and pull your shoulders back at the top of the spinal curl (two counts). Then, while maintaining your lower body position, put your hands together and reach out like you are diving (two counts). Bend your knees deeper and push out while reaching until your elbows are straight and behind your ears. Hold for four counts. Then place your hands on your knees for one more reach/scoop (as shown in Step 4) and proceed to Step 6.

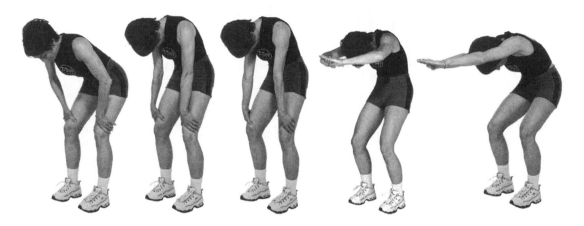

Step 6

Place your hands on the outside of your calves (not your ankles) and relax your upper body. While keeping your knees bent in KLT position, focus on releasing any tension in your neck or shoulders (especially the traps). You should feel the gravitational pull of your head relax and release any muscle tension. Now tighten your butt (feel those hamstrings) and push your hands into your calves at the same time you push your knees out and pull your shoulders back for leverage isometrics and spinal support.

Form Check If your hands are below your calves, you will not be able to optimize isometric activation of your lats.

Now gently rock your head four times without any other body movement and proceed to Step 7.

Step 7

Without releasing leverage isometric activation of your back muscles (from pushing in your calves while pushing out your knees and rolling your shoulders back), tuck your butt and curl your spine until your arms are straight. Then flip your palms forward and reach down with

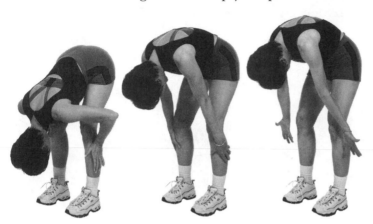

extended fingers as though your hands are extra-heavy. Tuck your butt at the same time as you reach down; you should feel an extra stretch in your mid- to lower back.

Step 8

Although Step 8 is really a continuation of Step 7, the reason I have it split into two parts is because I want to emphasize the importance of initiating the spinal roll-up with your shoulder and upper back muscles. Full fiber muscle activation of your latissimus dorsi and trapezius provide comprehensive spinal support as well as optimize thoracic activation and movement during roll-up. Continue reaching down as you roll up one vertebra at a time, keeping your hands alongside your body.

Form Check Keep your thumbs turned back as far as you can with your little fingers dragging along the sides of your thigh and in alignment with your hip joints. Do not lift your chin until the very end.

Step 9

Reach your shoulders up and back for a total of two shoulder rolls back.

Form Check Maintain lat activation and keep your hands below your waist or hips during shoulder roll. Keep your thumbs turned back as far as you can and really reach down to stretch your traps.

Now repeat the entire sequence, from Step 1 to Step 9.

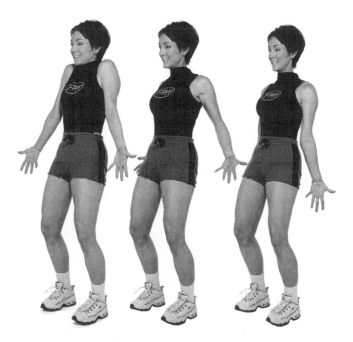

Step 10

Now reach your shoulders up and forward for a total of two shoulder rolls forward and finish with one more shoulder roll back, locking your lats with shoulders down.

Step 11

Interlock your hands together, tilt your shoulders back, and proceed to straighten your arms to the best of your ability.

Form Check Maintain your lower body position with your butt tucked under and your knees out in KLT. Your thumbnails, knuckles, and wrists should line up perfectly. As strength and flexibility improve, try to turn your elbows in, as shown in the photo. The focus is not so much on having your elbows completely straight but rather on keeping your shoulders back, turned out, and down.

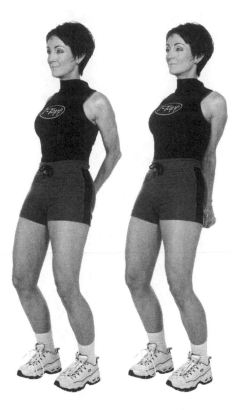

Now, with your arms as straight as possible and without release of shoulder position, inhale big and exhale bigger. You should feel your muscles stretching and your ribs expanding during the inhale, and you should feel your muscles tighten and your ribs pull in during the exhale.

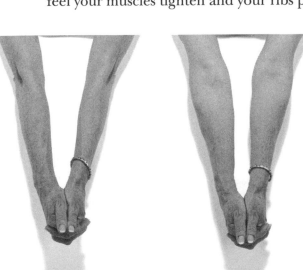

Form Check Concentrate on pulling your ribs all the way in during exhale until no air is left in your chest cavity.

Now lift and lower your arms four times without changing shoulder position, as shown in photo.

Alternative Position for Step 11 to Improve Shoulder Alignment

Instead of interlocking your hands, you can use a towel to optimize shoulder rotation. This not only works better for those who have special shoulder concerns (such as rotator cuff problems or frozen shoulder), but also works well for those who wish to intensify the effectiveness of Primary Back Stretch. When using a towel, it is important to start with your wrists in alignment with your shoulders. Then as you reach down, point your thumbs in toward your body and continue to rotate your thumbs out until they point to the sides (or to the best of your ability). For those who are more advanced, twist your elbows in to assist your shoulders to rotate out and your thumbs to rotate all the way back until they face the back wall. When using a towel, you should feel your chest open up, along with increased stretch of your pectoral

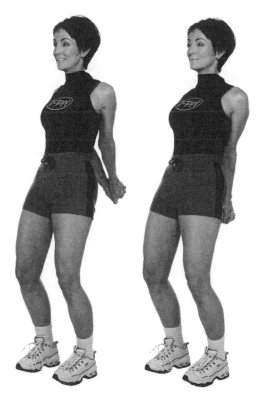

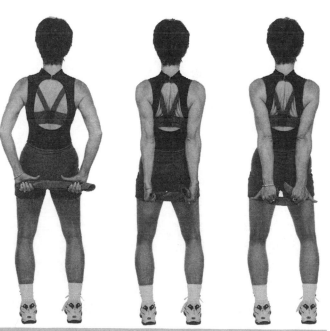

muscles. Using a towel also helps your body achieve optimal lymphatic flow during arm pumps.

MOST COMMON MISTAKES

Allowing your upper body to move while pumping your arms. This is not a large movement. Initially you may not be able to lift your arms as much as mine (as shown in photo), but even just a fraction of the movement delivers benefit.

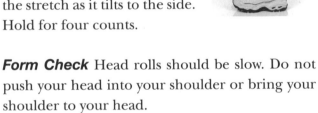

Step 12

While maintaining isometric isolation of your spine with correct shoulder, hip, and knee alignment, drop your chin and roll your head to your left. Let the weight of your head create the stretch as it tilts to the side. Hold for four counts.

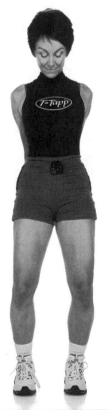

Form Check Head rolls should be slow. Do not push your head into your shoulder or bring your shoulder to your head.

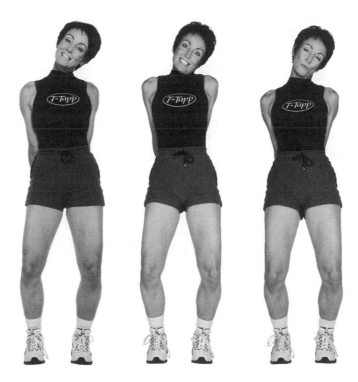

Step 13

Lift your shoulders as you inhale big. Then reach down with your hands to pull your shoulders down as you exhale bigger. Now roll your head back to center and continue to roll it to your right. Hold for four counts. Inhale big and exhale bigger. Repeat Steps 12 and 13.

Step 14

Before tilting your head to the right, it is important to reset your shoulder alignment by tightening the muscles between your shoulder blades. Hold for two counts. Next, tilt your head to the left for two counts. Then repeat head tilts to right and left for two counts each and return your head to center. Finish with four arm pumps.

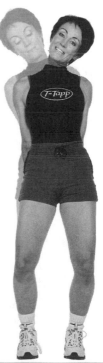

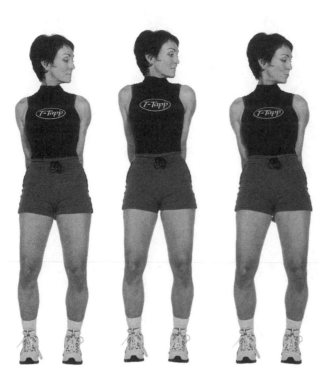

Step 15

Slowly turn your head as far to the left as you can, making sure to keep your shoulders back, butt tucked, and knees out in KLT (especially your right knee). Lift your shoulders up as you inhale big, and reach your hands and shoulders down as you exhale bigger. Now turn your head slowly to the right as far as you can without moving your body and with extra focus on keeping your left knee out in KLT. Again inhale big and exhale bigger.

Form Check Extra focus on keeping your butt tucked with knees out in KLT provides isometric support for your lower back, and keeping your shoulders back and down provides extra support for your neck.

Now repeat, turning your head to the left and then to the right without the inhale or exhale, holding four counts on each side. Repeat again with quicker movement, turning your head from left to right and holding two counts on each side, for two sets of two. Look forward and finish with four arm pumps.

MOST COMMON MISTAKE

Allowing your head to roll back can create strain on your neck; it is very important to keep your head straight.

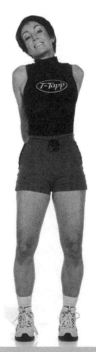

Step 16

Proceed to a flat back position, keeping your head level with your spine. Arch your butt to the ceiling and tighten. Use your lats and tighten the muscles between your shoulders to keep your shoulders back. Inhale and exhale.

Form Check Do not move your body as you lift your arms up and down four times.

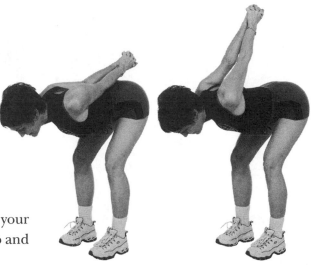

Step 17

Continue bending over for a full spinal stretch while maintaining the same arm position (with or without a towel) to your own personal max. Hold this position and tuck your chin as your inhale for one to two counts. You should feel increased stretching in your muscles throughout your torso and back. Then relax your head as you exhale for a full two counts. Repeat one more inhale/exhale with chin tucked on the inhale and with head relaxed on the exhale.

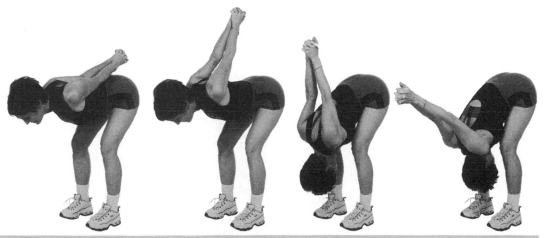

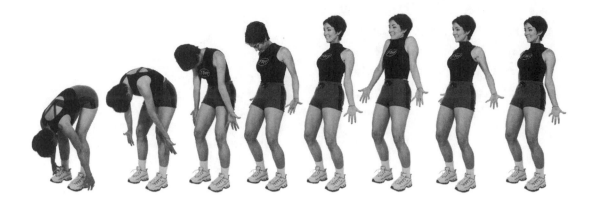

Step 18

Release your arms, flip your palms, and reach down as you tuck your butt and curl your back.

Form Check Use your lats and shoulder muscles to initiate a spinal roll.

Continue to tuck and pull your shoulders back as you roll up one vertebra at a time, bringing your chin up at the end. Finish with one big shoulder roll, up, back, and down.

You did it! Now take a water break.

Note: Since Primary Back Stretch is a very comprehensive exercise involving optimal lymphatic movement, you may feel a bit nauseated during your first spinal roll-up. Occurrence of this will depend on what you have consumed in the last twenty-four hours (you may feel it if you've consumed excessive sugar or alcohol), your recent level of inactivity, or the amount of medications you are taking.

PLIÉ SEQUENCE

I created the Plié Sequence for three reasons:

1. To increase cardiac conditioning
2. To provide simultaneous pumping of your upper and lower body lymph (your armpits and groin) zones for optimal lymphatic circulation and elimination, and
3. To improve left brain/right brain, mind/body coordination

In the beginning, it can be somewhat challenging to coordinate movement of your upper and lower body, but that's okay—you'll still achieve results if you're not able to do it perfectly. In fact, I suggest that you maintain isometric isolation of your lower body in a squat position during the first three segments (Crossover Head Pulls, Reverse Overhead Cross, and Jumping Jack Squats). Just focus on keeping your butt tucked with knees pushing out at all times to sustain optimal neurokinetic and lymphatic flow. Then, as you get more comfortable with the arm movements, try moving your legs at the same time without losing linear alignment. Spinal alignment from shoulder to hip is very important but very easy to lose until your upper back muscles develop enough isometric strength to hold your shoulders back without losing lower back muscle activation. Maintaining this alignment not only empowers your body to burn fat at a premium, it also develops body-sculpting inch loss in your arms, legs, back, and belly.

Although all T-Tapp movements are comprehensive and compound, enabling your body to target all areas of concern, I believe that Plié Sequence is the most effective at burning back fat. So let's get started and burn some fat for fuel!

Step 1

Plant your feet shoulder width apart with toes turned out at a 30-degree angle or less. Distance of stance can vary from one person to another, but your shoulders should be in alignment with or inside your heels. It

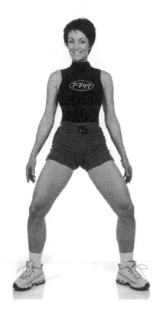

is important to apply the primary principles of T-Tapp at all times (shoulders back, butt tucked, and knees out in KLT). Once the muscles in your back become stronger and more flexible, it's okay to have a wider stance as long as you can maintain these primary principles. Now press the tips of all your fingers onto your thumb to make the shape of an O. I call this the doughnut hand position—it increases nerve stimulus for optimal neurokinetic flow without increase of lactic acid. Feel the difference as opposed to when you use a clenched fist? The doughnut hand position is especially helpful for those who have internal inflammation conditions like arthritis or fibromyalgia.

Step 2: Crossover Head Pulls

Maintain your upper body position with shoulders back and butt tucked as you reach down with your arms (count one, crossing them in front of your chest, and then bringing them all the way up above your head and behind your ears, as shown in the first three images).

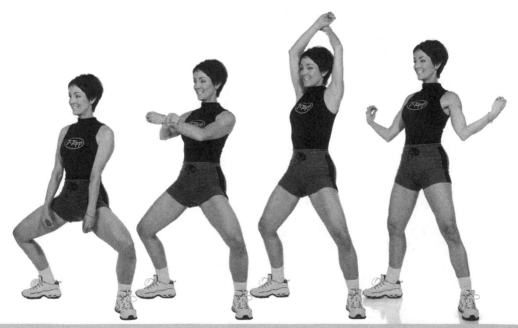

Form Check Keep pushing your knees out and tucking your butt as you straighten your legs.

Now pull your arms down into a wide W position (count two) with elbows forward and hands back—both aligned with your shoulders and behind your ears. Your palms should be facing the center of your body. Your butt should still be tucked and your knees nearly straight, but still turned out in KLT position.

MOST COMMON MISTAKES

Allowing your shoulders to come forward in front of your hips during arm movements releases the activation of your upper back muscles, especially the lats. Bringing your shoulders forward creates an automatic release of the abdominal, lower back, and gluteal muscles, too, so use your lats to keep those shoulders back!

Another common mistake is completely straightening your knees and relaxing your thighs at the top of the plié movement. *Tip:* Try turning out your knee as you straighten your legs to maintain muscle activation from your hip joint to your knee.

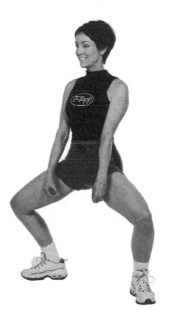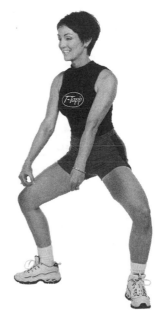

Step 3: Reverse Overhead Cross

Start bending your knees as you bring your arms back up and down in front of your chest without releasing shoulder alignment. Your lower body should be in the lowest plié position by count three with your arms out to the sides. Continue moving your arms straight up in alignment with your shoulders until they are by your ears (count four). Your doughnut hand position should flip up once your arms lift above your shoulders.

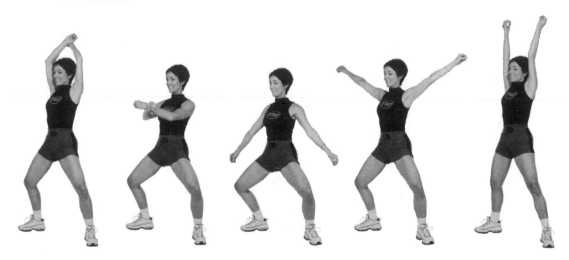

Form Check Keep tightening your lats, tucking your butt, and pushing your knees out at all times. Keep your elbows straight and your butt tucked when your arms are all the way up, too.

MOST COMMON MISTAKE

Release of butt, hands in front of ears, and bent elbows inactivate muscle attachments in your back, arms, and stomach. Even though the second photo shows that my butt is tucked, the straight arms in front of the ears create an imbalance of muscle activation between my shoulder and back muscles. *Tip:* Tuck your butt even more and really reach your arms up to maintain activation of the muscles along your spine.

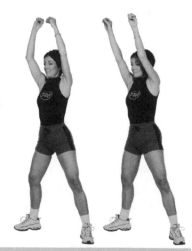

Repeat Steps 2 and 3 for a total of eight repetitions, four counts each. Count as follows: hands are down in front (count one), arms are in W position (count two), hands are back down (count three), arms are all the way up (count four).

Note: there is a bit of a swing to this movement, but do not go too fast. The most important factor is to never, ever release your upper back muscles, especially your lats. And as always, keep your butt tucked.

Proceed to Step 4 without stopping.

Step 4: Jumping Jack Squats

Push your knees out and pull your arms down into a big W while lowering your body into a plié squat position (count one).

Form Check In addition to keeping your shoulders back, butt tucked, and knees in KLT, push your elbows forward and pull your hands back with palms facing center. This push/pull action will help you maintain correct linear alignment of your wrists and elbows with your shoulders.

Then straighten your knees as you punch your arms up with a twist of the wrist so that your palms face forward (count two).

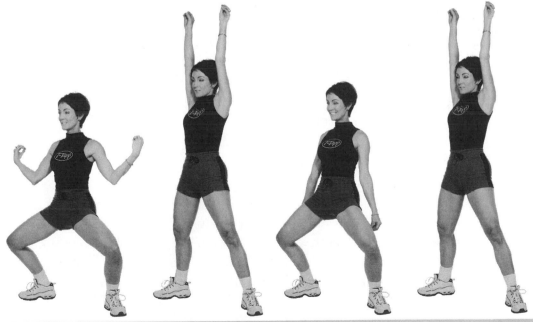

Form Check In addition to keeping your arms straight with wrists and shoulders in alignment, do not relax your thighs or release your butt tuck. In fact, your arms should feel like they're reaching up behind your ears.

Now quickly bring your straight arms down (count three) and back up (count four) without losing linear alignment. When executing optimal form, your arms should feel like they are reaching away during counts three and four.

MOST COMMON MISTAKES

Elbows back and hands too high do not allow your back muscles to fully contract, especially your lats and obliques. Furthermore, hands in front with elbows back will cause your shoulders to pronate during movement. This can cause you to develop muscle imbalance between your traps and lats.

Arms in front of ears, when above your head, inactivate your upper back and shoulder muscles as well as your butt tuck. If you don't keep your arms back behind your ears and in alignment with your shoulders during counts three and four, your body can develop muscle imbalance or muscle strain. _Tip:_ To help your body maintain correct alignment and isometric contractions, do not go too fast.

Repeat for a total of eight repetitions, four counts each. Count as follows: pull arms into W (count one), punch arms up (count two), straight arms down (count three), and straight arms up (count four).

Note: After finishing your eighth repetition, instead of again pulling your arms into a W position, stop when your elbows are level with your shoulders. Your wrists should be in alignment with your elbows with palms facing center, and your lower body should be in a moderate squat with your butt tucked and knees out. Hold this position for two counts while you inhale and exhale, then proceed to Step 5.

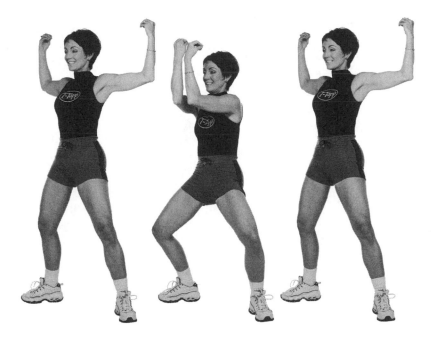

Step 5: Chest Press
Maintain elbow/shoulder and elbow/wrist alignment as you bring your elbows forward to the center of your body.

Form Check Do not release your shoulders as your elbows press forward—keep your lats tight. Your elbows should feel like they are pressing against a weight.

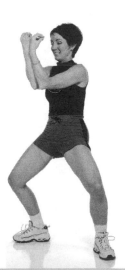

Continue to maintain this alignment while you move your elbows all the way back behind your ears.

MOST COMMON MISTAKES
When elbows drop below (or rise above) shoulder alignment, your body loses full fiber activation of several muscles, especially your pecs and lats.

Dropping your elbows below your shoulders while behind your ears is not only the most common but also the easiest mistake to make without realizing it. That's because even the slightest drop will affect results. Look closely at the two photos—see how, in the right image, my elbows are only an inch or two lower than my shoulders and slightly in front of my ears? That little inch off alignment makes a big difference in receiving results!

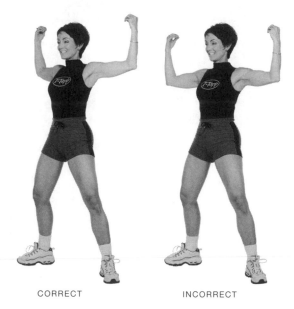

CORRECT   INCORRECT

Repeat for a total of eight repetitions. Each repetition is counted as follows: elbows forward (counts one and two), elbows out (counts three and four).

Proceed to Step 6 without stopping.

Step 6: Chest Press Combo

Tuck butt and bend your knees deep in KLT as you punch your arms up with a twist of the wrist so your palms face forward.

Form Check Maintain alignment of your wrists to your shoulders and do not relax your thighs or release your butt tuck.

Then straighten your knees as you pull your elbows down, stopping at shoulder level.

Form Check Along with having your elbows back behind your ears, concentrate on tightening your back muscles at the point when your elbows become level with your shoulders. This little isometric contraction will assist your body not only to maintain correct alignment, but also to optimize lymphatic flow.

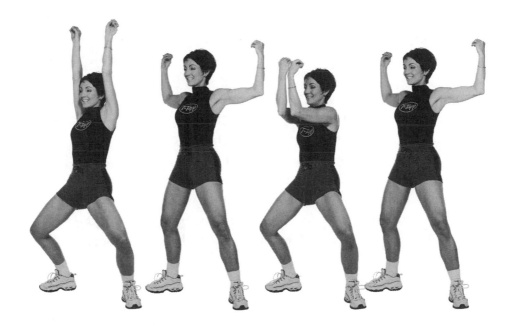

Then bring your elbows forward to the center of your body and open them all the way back behind your ears without losing alignment with your shoulders.

Form Check Retighten your back muscles again once your elbows are all the way behind your ears.

Repeat this sequence for a total of eight repetitions. Count as follows: arms up (counts one and two), elbows down to shoulders (counts three and four), elbows forward (counts five and six), elbows out (counts seven and eight).

REACH SCOOPS

I created Reach Scoops to be done after the Plié Sequence to provide lateral stretching for your spine and to help your body slowly lower its heart rate. With every tuck, reach, and scoop this exercise will help your body increase its stretch capacity from rib to hip, allowing your torso muscles to better cinch in, uplift, tighten, and tone. Reach Scoops also create comprehensive and compound activation of your abdominal muscles with every simultaneous KLT push. So, focus on form—you'll see and feel the difference with Reach Scoops.

All Steps

It is important to hold your body in the following position during the first inhale/exhale to control your body's heart rate so it can slow down gradually. With left arm up and behind your ear, the weight of your body should be on your right leg with your butt tucked and right knee out. Your upper body should be slightly tilted to the right and your right shoulder should be in lateral alignment with your right hip. Your right arm should be relaxed and hanging straight down. Inhale big and exhale bigger (two counts each).

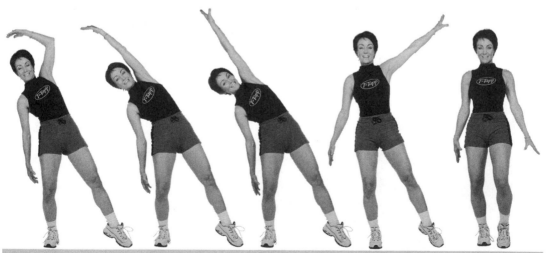

Repeat the inhale, but this time tilt your upper body over more and reach with your left arm until your elbow straightens (two counts).

Form Check Tuck your butt and push your right knee out at same time you reach over to your personal max. *Tip:* Reach your right hand down at the same time you are reaching overhead with your left arm. When doing so you should feel an extended stretch from rib to hip on the left side of your body.

Then while exhaling, flip your left palm, reaching up and out with it until your body returns to an upright position with your left arm down along your side (two counts).

Form Check Tuck your butt and push your right knee out at the same time you flip, reach, and scoop. You should feel additional tightening in your lower tummy (the transverse abdominus muscle). At the same time your left arm is moving, bring your left foot in and tap the floor for extra lymphatic benefit.

Now repeat to other side with your right arm up and your left leg supporting the weight of your body.

MOST COMMON MISTAKES

Allowing one shoulder to tilt back and/or allowing your reach/ scoop arm to reach in front of your ear are common mistakes. That's because our spines do not use lateral movements in daily activity. Maintaining linear alignment (shoulder to shoulder and shoulder to hip) is important not only for results, but also for balanced muscle stretching as well as development. You should feel the muscles in your tummy and torso tighten with every tuck, reach, and scoop. Another common mistake is allowing your hand to touch your thigh. Let the weight of your arm add to the weight of your body during the tilt. This will maximize activation of your muscles (comprehensive and compound) so your body can build a better muscle girdle.

Repeat for a total of eight repetitions, alternating each side (left/right count one, left/right count two, etc.) while breathing normally.

JAZZ TWIST

Jazz Twists are designed to stretch and release muscle tension between your shoulder blades and target lymph nodes in the middle of your back (and your thoracic duct), as well as help your body continue to lower its heart rate. Twisting your spine in linear alignment in Jazz Twist, after laterally bending and stretching it during Reach Scoops, not only helps you control your heart rate, but also helps your body develop a stronger, more flexible spine. Furthermore, twisting your upper spine while maintaining isometric isolation of your lower spine also optimizes lymphatic function. But don't forget to keep your butt tucked and your back straight with hips and shoulders in alignment! Linear alignment and isometric isolation are what makes this exercise different from a traditional jazz movement.

All Steps

Place your left arm at shoulder height with fingers pulled back, elbow straight, and shoulders back and in alignment with your hips. Your right hand should be below your waist with your thumb pushing into your back. This not only helps pull your right shoulder back, it also

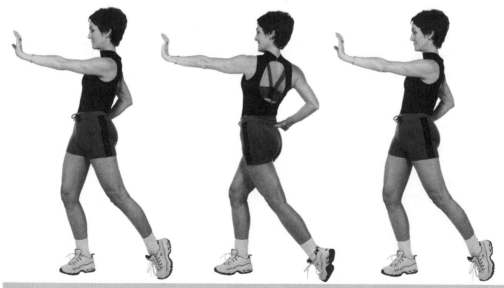

helps your body sustain isometric activation of the muscles in your back during movement. Now tuck your butt and push your right knee out into KLT position. Inhale and exhale. Inhale again, but during this exhale pull your right shoulder back and reach out with your left hand, twisting your upper body as much as you can. Ultimately, the body position you are trying to achieve is similar to an archery pull, where your left wrist and your left and right shoulders are in a straight line. Once you have achieved this position to the best of your ability, inhale and exhale again and hold for four counts. As you inhale you should feel your muscles stretch all the way down your spine, and during the exhale you should feel your muscles pull your ribs together. Now pull your left shoulder back, without bending your elbow or shifting alignment, until your body is back in the starting position.

Form Check Push your thumb and tuck your butt during the exhale to increase the intensity of isometric contraction.

MOST COMMON MISTAKES

Allowing your upper body to tilt forward in front of your hip not only releases your butt tuck, which causes inactivation of your lower back and abdominal muscles, but also creates an imbalance of muscle development. Another common mistake is allowing your left arm to move across your body instead of staying in alignment with your left shoulder.

Repeat Jazz Twist "stretch" to other side, using your right arm at shoulder height. Then repeat Jazz Twist with movement as follows: reach and pull right shoulder back four times (one count each), reach and pull left shoulder back four times (one count each). Then repeat two times on each side, for a total of two sets of two.

Form Check This movement is done with a bit of momentum, but do not forget to keep tucking your butt and keep your knee out in KLT at all times.

Proceed to The Box.

THE BOX

Although visually similar to other waist-bending, torso-trimming exercises, The Box is much more comprehensive and therefore more effective in flattening your stomach, as well as trimming your torso. Maintaining isolation of your lower body with tucked butt and KLT along with maintaining linear alignment of your shoulder to hip during The Box enables your body to maximize muscle mechanics. Furthermore, stabilization of your lower body while bending your upper spine to the front, side, and back assists lymphatic function and improves spinal strength and flexibility. Last of all, the use of leverage isometrics while you manually help your body reposition internal organs during movement helps your abdominal muscles develop girdle density to flatten your lower tummy and cinch your waist.

Step 1

Assume the T-Tapp stance and place your hands below your waist with thumbs pushing into your back. In addition to pushing your thumbs, pull your fingers off your body and keep your elbows back. By doing so you should feel increased activation of the muscles in your back and between your shoulder blades. Remember, the secret to a flat stomach is linear alignment of your shoulder to hip.

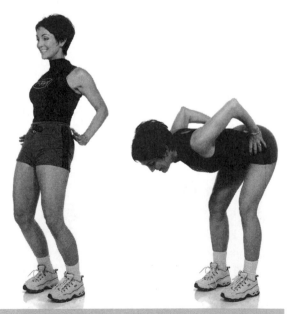

Now bend at your waist until your shoulders are level with your hips. Keep pushing with your thumbs for leverage isometrics and to help keep your elbows up toward the ceiling. Now slightly move your flat back up and down four times.

Form Check Arch your butt to the ceiling as you bend into flat back position to comprehensively activate your lower back, abdominal, and hamstring muscles.

Step 2

Do what I call putting your organs in place by pushing both of your hands into your lower abdominal cavity. You should feel your internal organs—including your bladder and intestines—shift up. Keep pressing your hands in and up as you straighten your upper body until your shoulders are back and aligned with your hips.

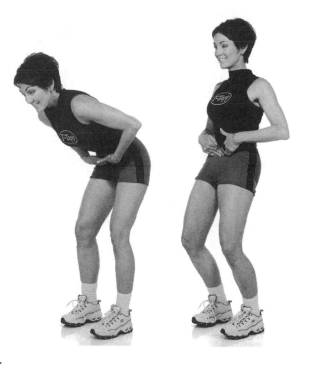

Form Check Knees should be bent and pushing out at all times to maintain activation of your abdominal muscles, especially the transverse abdominus.

Step 3

Tilt your upper body to the right while maintaining lower-body isolation in the T-Tapp stance. With an additional contraction, tighten your tucked butt and push your left knee out as you pull your upper body into an upright position. Repeat for a total of four tilts (one count each) to your right.

Form Check You should feel your internal core and abdominal muscles tighten when you tighten, tuck, push, and pull. If not, don't worry—neuro-kinetic connection does improve with time. In fact, that's one of the reasons why you keep pressing your hands just below your navel while tilting. This pressure not only helps your body main-

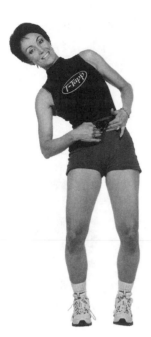
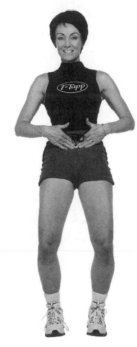

tain better isometric activation of the muscles in your torso (lats and obliques), it also allows stronger nerve transmission to occur at the point where your hands are pressing in. This, in turn, enables your body to develop faster neurokinetic connection to your muscles when needed. Plus it's easier for your abdominal muscles to shorten their fibers and cinch in when internal organs aren't pressing out! Eventually your muscles will be able to hold those organs in without manual assistance.

MOST COMMON MISTAKES

Allowing your shoulders to tilt back instead of keeping your shoulders square will cause your body to lose comprehensive activation of the muscles in your upper back and shoulders. Allowing your lower body to shift weight will cause you to lose proper hip, knee, and ankle alignment. Lower body stabilization is important for your body to create long, lean muscle development. That's because when your lower body shifts out of alignment it creates isotonic rather than isometric movement, and isotonic muscle movement can cause your waist to thicken!

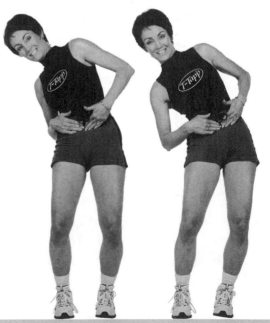

Step 4

Now slightly pulse your shoulders and upper body back four times (one count each) without losing isolation of your lower body in the T-Tapp stance. During this step you are primarily resetting your shoulders to release muscle tension in your shoulders and neck, as well as assist lymphatic function.

MOST COMMON MISTAKE

Leaning too far back and pushing your pelvic/hip area too far forward are easy to do if you use momentum to tilt. *Tip:* Pushing your thumbs in your back each time you reset your shoulders will help prevent lower body movement.

Step 5

Repeat Step 2 and put your organs in place.

Step 6

Repeat upper body tilts to your left for a total of four repetitions (one count each).

Repeat entire box sequence with two repetitions on each side—front, right side, back, and left side—but this time keep your hands below your waist with your thumbs pushing into your body to optimize activation of your lats and oblique muscles.

Proceed to Oil Wells without stopping.

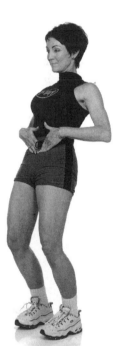

OIL WELLS

Oil Wells are designed to help your body release lower back tension as well as help strengthen your lower back and abdominal muscles. As always, focus on form to reap these rewards. Knees out to KLT feels so good during Oil Wells, especially for those who have existing back issues. This little exercise also helps improve strength and flexibility in your upper back and shoulder muscles.

Starting Position

Place your feet shoulder width apart with toes forward and knees bent pushing out into KLT. Your hands should be together in a dive position.

Assume a flat back position with your shoulders and back level with your hips and with your butt arching up toward the ceiling (not tucked). You should feel like your back is scooping out.

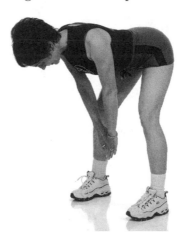

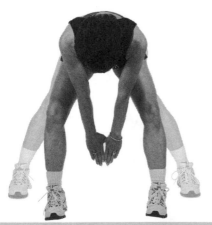

MOST COMMON MISTAKE

Having too wide a stance will alter your ability to maintain activation of your abdominal muscles, especially the transverse abdominus. It is important to maintain knee-to-ankle linear alignment at all times.

Step 1

Keep your butt arching up and your knees pushing out as you reach between your legs with your arms straight and hands together (count one). Return to a flat back position (count two), but continue your arm movement up and back for a full shoulder roll (counts three and four).

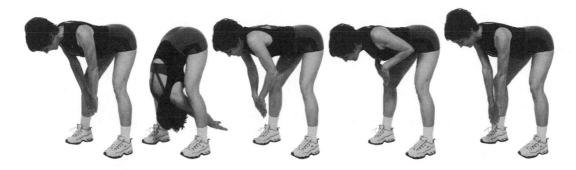

Form Check Keep your lats tight during your shoulder roll and when your arms reach down. *Tip:* Pull your shoulders back when reaching your arms down. Additionally, your head should stay relaxed and your hands should stay together while reaching through your legs.

MOST COMMON MISTAKE

Releasing your shoulders after the shoulder roll inactivates your back and abdominal muscles.

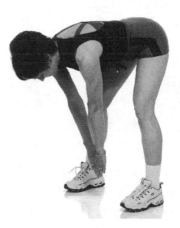

Repeat Oil Wells for a total of eight repetitions (four counts each).

Step 2

While maintaining your lower body in T-Tapp stance and your hands together in dive position, reach down as you tuck your butt and slowly roll up one vertebra at a time as shown in first three images (four counts). Lift your head and then your arms with bent elbows and hands together and finish your spinal roll with four arm pumps above your head (four counts).

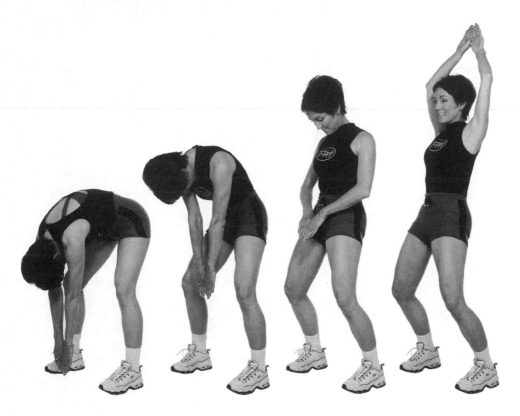

Form Check Keep your back muscles tight to help stabilize your shoulders every time you pull your hands back. It's important to keep your butt tucked and knees out too.

Repeat Steps 1 and 2, Oil Wells and spinal roll-up.

Step 3

Relax your head but keep your back muscles tight by pushing your hands on the outside of your legs below your knees. As always, keep your knees bent in KLT position. Now gently rock your head four times without moving your body.

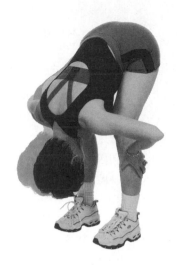

Step 4

Finish with one final spinal roll-up and a big shoulder roll.

Proceed to T-Tapp Twist/Pull the Weeds without stopping, or take a water break if needed.

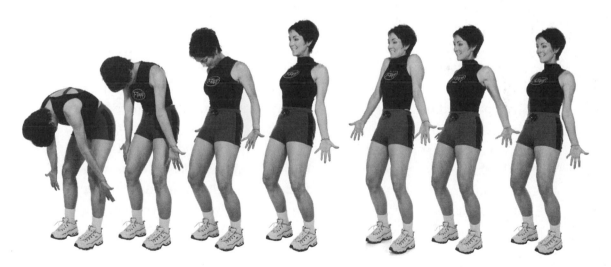

T-TAPP TWIST/PULL THE WEEDS

I consider T-Tapp Twist/Pull the Weeds to be one of my signature movements, but it should never be done without first doing Primary Back Stretch to properly warm up your spine. Its comprehensive design helps your body help itself in so many ways—both in fitness and in health. Twisting your upper body while maintaining isolation of your lower body with the T-Tapp stance helps your body develop spinal strength and flexibility, optimize lymphatic flow, increase circulation, and accelerate inch loss from muscle density development. Even if you did nothing but Primary Back Stretch and T-Tapp Twist/Pull the Weeds, you would see a trimmer torso and a flatter tummy within days.

T-Tapp Twist especially targets the thoracic area of your spine (the middle of your back)—an area that is often overlooked and underused during daily activity. But remember, developing muscles with strength and flexibility takes time, so it is important to focus on form while performing this move. Don't worry if you cannot bend or twist as far as I do in the photos—just do it to the best of your ability, and you will receive the same benefits. T-Tapp Twist, like all T-Tapp exercises, is designed to be progressive, which means that one never achieves perfect form. Going to your personal max during comprehensive, compound muscle movement allows your muscles to be continuously challenged, so there's never a need to increase repetitions or add weight. In fact, it is better to do fewer repetitions to the best of your ability with T-Tapp Twist than to execute eight repetitions without focus. Discover how linear isometric isolation of your spine in combination with large muscle movement enables your body to optimize function and receive results faster with T-Tapp Twist/Pull the Weeds.

Starting Position

Place your feet approximately twelve inches apart or less with toes forward, knees bent and pushing out, butt tucked, and shoulders back and in alignment with your hips. *It is very important to hold this position at*

all times during T-Tapp Twist.
A stance that is too wide
makes it more difficult to
create full fiber activation
of the muscles that attach
from your lower spine to
your hip. Comprehensive,
compound activation of
these muscles not only
helps to protect your spine,
but also helps your body develop muscles with greater
girdle density so you can
lose inches quicker. It is better to have a stance that is
too narrow than too wide.

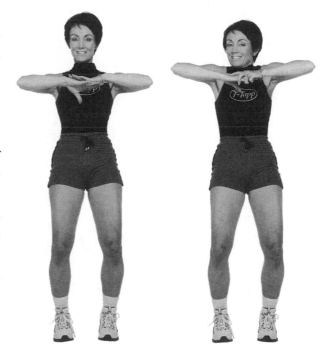

Now place your arms
just below your collarbone
with elbows level and in alignment with your shoulders. It is important
to establish full fiber activation of your upper back and shoulder muscles, too, especially the latissimus dorsi and trapezius. Let your shoulders rise as you inhale big, then pull your shoulders back and down
while you exhale. You should feel a deep stretch within your neck
(trapezius) as well as deep isometric activation of your muscles along
the sides of your back and shoulders (lats).

Form Check Press your hands on top of each other and try to maintain
pressure between them during this exercise. This will help your body
create balanced isometric activation of your lat and oblique muscles,
especially when twisting and during spinal roll-up.

Step 1: Tuck and Twist/Spinal Stretch

Inhale big again, but during this exhale twist your upper body to the left as far as you can (look at your left elbow) without changing your lower body position. Hold for four counts. Then relax your spinal stretch just a little bit (look over your hands), but do not release your butt tuck. Inhale again, but during this exhale, increase the intensity of your butt tuck and push your right knee out to your personal max while looking at your left elbow and reaching back as far as you can. Hold for four counts. Then inhale big (two counts) and exhale bigger (two counts) to maximize stretch and lymphatic function.

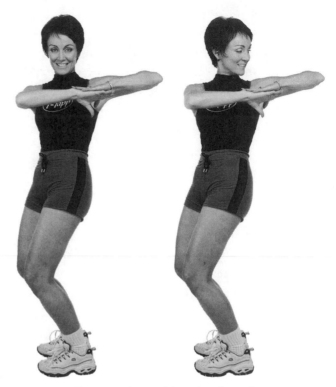

Repeat to the right side.

Form Check Really focus on maintaining perfect alignment of your right elbow to shoulder when reaching back. However, notice in the photo how my front elbow is slightly lower? It's okay to let your front elbow drop when you twist your upper body to the back. In fact, it can help you establish better comprehensive contraction in your lat and trap muscles. It also helps release muscle tension along your neck, especially in the traps. But never allow your reaching elbow to drop lower than your shoulder!

Return to starting position and proceed to Step 2.

Step 2

Twist your upper body to the right and pulse for two counts without moving your lower body. In fact, while twisting to the right, focus on tightening your left knee and thigh to help keep it out and not move inward. You might not be able to twist as far back, but the object is to isolate your lower body from your upper body while twisting. Do not shift your weight; just twist your upper spine.

Form Check Look at your elbow with your eyes during twist for optimal stretch of your spine all the way up through your neck (cervical vertebrae).

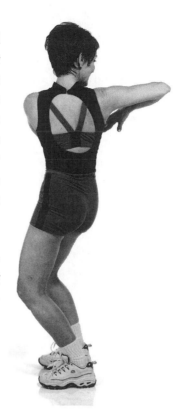

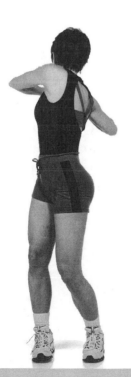

MOST COMMON MISTAKES

Releasing your knee inward during the upper body twist, allowing your reaching elbow to drop lower than your shoulder, and not keeping your butt tucked can create unsafe conditions for your spine and lessen the effectiveness of this exercise.

Step 3

Now twist all the way over to your left side in one count until your shoulders are square to the side. Did you tuck, tighten, and push out with your right knee and thigh while twisting? Continue to tighten your tuck and push your right knee out as you reach down with your upper body with your hands aiming toward your ankle or to the back of your heel.

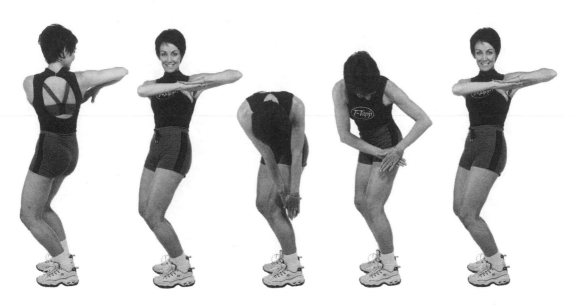

Form Check Your shoulders should be level and your head relaxed without tension in your neck. Weight distribution should be equal or slightly more on your left leg when reaching down. Now slowly roll back up one vertebra at a time, keeping your upper body in a spinal twist position (four counts). Keep tucking and pushing KLT all the time during your spinal roll-up, and do not lift your head until count four.

Form Check Your upper body should be facing to the side and your lower body should be facing to the front on count four.

MOST COMMON MISTAKE

Do not shift your weight when reaching down. The object is not how far down you can reach, but how well you can achieve correct form while reaching down. As you can see from my image on the left, I am only able to reach to the middle of my thigh when executing correct form. My image on the right shows me shifting my weight so I can reach further, but it decreases my ability to lose inches.

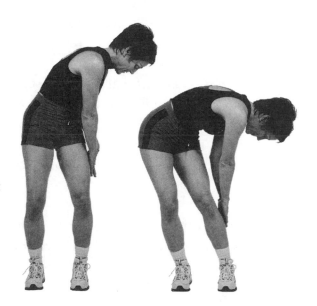

Ability to Reach Based on Body Type

In addition to spinal strength and flexibility, your body type (length of spine) will also determine how far down you can reach. Long Torso/Short Leg body types, like me, should aim behind their knee and reach to the top of their calf muscle. Combo body types, as shown

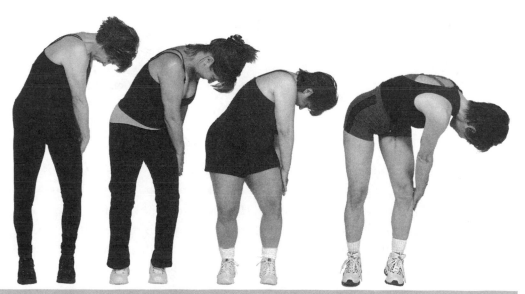

by the two middle images, have less length from rib to hip, so they will not be able to reach quite as far. If you have a Combo–borderline Long Torso (second image from right), you should aim behind, but reach to the top of your knee; if you have a Combo–borderline Short Torso, you should aim behind your knee and reach the middle of your thigh. If you have a Short Torso/Long Leg body type, you should focus on twisting to the best of your ability without releasing your butt tuck and aim just below your hip or the top of your thigh (as shown in photo, left image)

Form Check Regardless of body type, concentrate on maintaining your spinal twist throughout the entire roll-up and be sure to push out your opposite knee (KLT) to maintain isometric isolation of your lower back and hips.

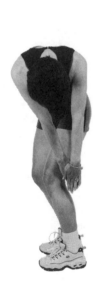 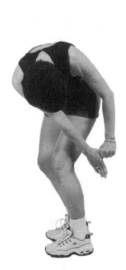 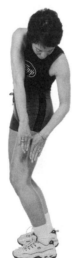

MOST COMMON MISTAKE

Another common mistake when reaching down is having one shoulder higher than the other. Try to keep your shoulders level at all times. *Tip:* Pull on your extended arm when reaching down and while rolling up to help your body achieve optimal spinal twist with level shoulders.

Repeat for a total of eight repetitions, eight counts each, each repetition counted as follows: twist to the right for two, over to the left in one (count three), then reach down (count four) and roll it back up (counts five to eight). On the eighth repetition, do not roll back up—instead of rolling up during counts five through eight, move your body from side to front in a flat back position (counts five, six, and seven) and finish by pulling your shoulders back (count eight). You are now ready to continue with the next set of movements, called Pull the Weeds.

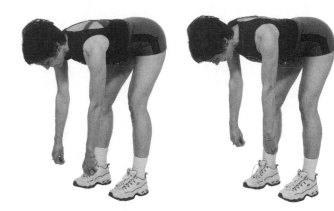

Step 4: Pull the Weeds

Pull your elbows up level to your shoulders or a little higher, toward your ears and aiming forward to the front wall as you pull up (count one). Your wrists should be in alignment with your elbows and your lower body should remain in the T-Tapp stance. Now punch your arms straight down, but don't release your shoulders (count two). Your elbows should be straight with wrists in linear alignment with your shoulders. Do not cross your wrists.

Form Check Tighten your lats to keep your shoulders back, and arch your butt up toward the ceiling at all times to isometrically secure your back and abdominal area. Only your arms should move.

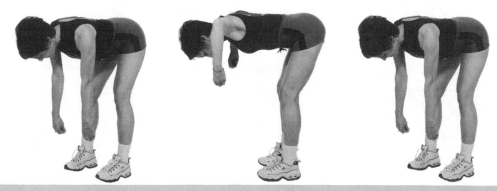

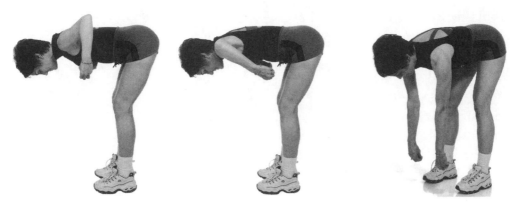

MOST COMMON MISTAKES

Pulling your elbows back behind your shoulders releases your triceps and lat muscles. Allowing your wrists to aim back and out of alignment with your elbows will pronate your shoulders. Releasing your shoulders when punching down inactivates upper back and abdominal muscles.

Repeat for a total of eight repetitions, two counts each. Finish with two head rocks, one spinal roll-up, and one shoulder roll.

Repeat entire T-Tapp Twist/Pull the Weeds sequence on the opposite side, ending with another set of two head rocks, one spinal roll-up and one shoulder roll. Now take a water break before proceeding to Hoe Downs.

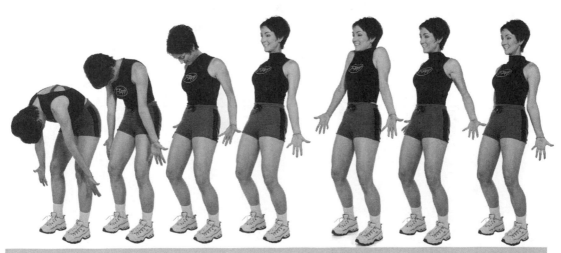

HOE DOWNS

Can minimal movement deliver maximum results? It can with Hoe Downs! I created this deceptively simple little exercise to comprehensively deliver a multitude of mental, physical, and health benefits. It may look easy, but within three minutes, regardless of age or fitness level, you will be breathing hard, your heart rate will increase, and your energy level will soar. I consider Hoe Downs to be the ultimate mini-max move, a little move that delivers big results.

That's because Hoe Downs incorporate comprehensive, compound large muscle movement along with isometric linear alignment and lymphatic pumping with every knee lift and floor tap. Nearly twenty years ago, I discovered that the combination of these factors can significantly increase cardiovascular rate, which is why all T-Tapp exercises are aerobic—especially Hoe Downs.

What's more, Hoe Downs involve simultaneous left-brain/right-brain cognitive processing for optimal brain balance. From the start, coordination can be challenging, especially when doing single-count sets, but every time you do Hoe Downs, your brain-to-body transmission will improve. In fact, recent research has revealed how important it is to exercise the brain as well as the body for quality of life in our senior years.

Additionally, Hoe Downs work well to offset stress, help blast the blues away, and increase mental clarity. Hoe Downs can also help control hormonal mood swings often associated with PMS and menopause.

Best of all, Hoe Downs work wonders in helping your body control blood sugar. Whether you're dealing with a diabetic condition or just want to burn excess glucose before it converts to fat, Hoe Downs work—and they work fast. Informal tests have revealed that glucose levels drop an average of 62 to 85 points with just one set of Hoe Downs after a meal or snack!

Hoe Downs are easy, fast, and can be done anywhere. They're the perfect example of how less *is* more with T-Tapp!

Starting Position

Assume the T-Tapp stance but shift your weight to your left leg. Your left knee should be bent in KLT position, your butt tucked, and your right toe on the floor. Keep your shoulders back in alignment with your hips while you extend your hands out to the sides of your body with palms up and your thumbs back. Now push your elbows forward and pull your hands back. You should feel your shoulders pull back and every muscle in your upper back tighten.

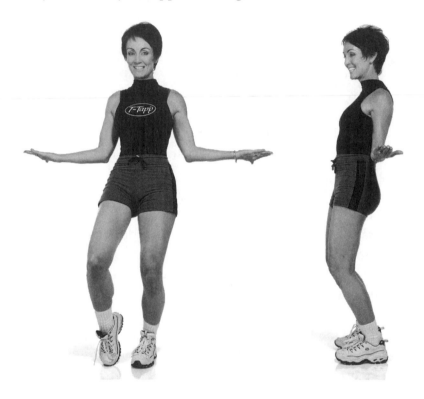

Form Check Linear alignment is very important. Your elbows and palms should be level. Your shoulders, elbows, and wrists should be in alignment. Your butt should be tucked with knees out toward little toes and your hips should be in alignment with your shoulders.

Now that every muscle in your body is isometrically activated, let's get started. Inhale big, exhale bigger and pull your shoulders down.

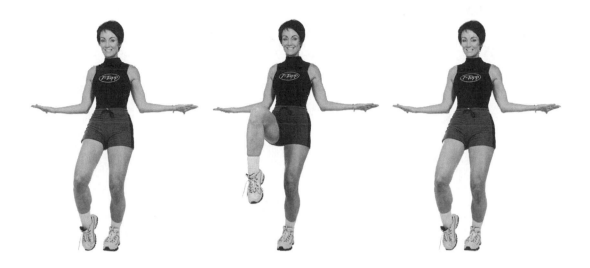

Step 1

Inhale big, and during the exhale, pull your shoulders down. Lift your right knee up in alignment with your right shoulder (count one) and then tap your toes to the floor (count two). Repeat for a total of four lift/taps (eight counts).

Form Check Keep your shoulders back, butt tucked, and left knee bent in KLT at all times.

MOST COMMON MISTAKE

Moving your upper body forward as you lift your knee or allowing your knee to lift to the center of your body instead of aiming at your shoulder are common mistakes. When your knee aims to the center of your body, you inactivate abdominal muscles. *Tip:* Tighten the muscles between your shoulder blades and tuck your butt every time you lift your knee. This will help stabilize your spine and deliver faster inch loss in your tummy.

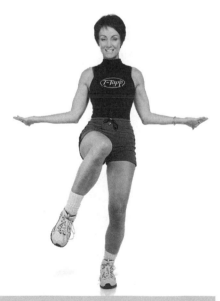

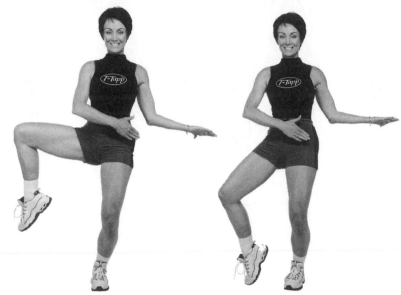

Step 2

Without stopping, lift your right knee up and out to the right side as you bring your right hand across your body to the left (count one) and tap your toes to the floor (count two). Repeat for a total of four lift/taps (eight counts).

Form Check Linear alignment is important during the lift/tap movement. In addition to aiming your knee toward the shoulder while lifting, also keep your foot pointed and in alignment with your knee. *Tip:* Pointing your toe intensifies activation of abdominal muscles.

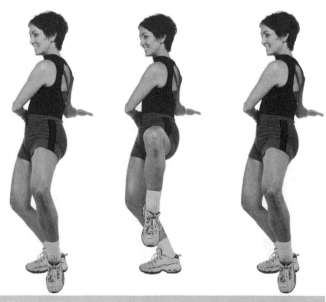

MOST COMMON MISTAKES

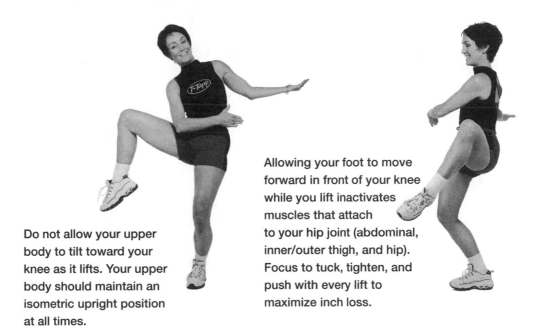

Do not allow your upper body to tilt toward your knee as it lifts. Your upper body should maintain an isometric upright position at all times.

Allowing your foot to move forward in front of your knee while you lift inactivates muscles that attach to your hip joint (abdominal, inner/outer thigh, and hip). Focus to tuck, tighten, and push with every lift to maximize inch loss.

Repeat steps one and two as follows: two sets of four lift/taps (eight counts front/eight counts on the right side, twice), two sets of two lift/taps (counts one to four front/five to eight right side, twice), and one set of four single lift/taps (counts one and two front/three and four right side, four times), all without stopping.

Then while inhaling and exhaling, do one shoulder roll and reset to the starting position to repeat the same sequence on the other side (two sets of four, two sets of two, and one set of four single lift/taps with left knee).

Then inhale big, exhale bigger, and repeat the entire sequence (right, then left) for a total of two sets of Hoe Downs.

YOU DID IT!

You did it! Now take a water break and *have a great day.*
This concludes your fifteen-minute T-Tapp
Basic Plus Workout. Or if you wish, you can continue
on to the next chapter for more core challenge
and body sculpting movements from the
T-Tapp Total Workout

The T-Tapp Total Workout

The first fifteen minutes of the T-Tapp Total Workout is the Basic Plus Workout sequence found in Chapter 4. While Basic Plus provides dramatic inch loss and boosts feelings of well-being, this Total Workout takes all of that to the next level.

These additional thirty minutes of exercises really concentrate on the core, delivering increased strength and flexibility and promoting better balance. From start to finish, the Total Workout will sculpt your muscles, strengthen your center, and speed up your metabolism so that you will see results—fast.

LUNGE SEQUENCE

Most people use traditional lunges to trim and tone their thighs, but when you apply T-Tapp techniques, lunges become much more effective. The Lunge Sequence is designed to comprehensively fatigue all of your thigh muscles so you develop muscle density instead of bulk for long, lean legs. Furthermore, the sequence of T-Tapp Lunges is designed to progressively prepare your body to use more of its intrinsic and core muscles during the Balance Sequence and Thread the Needle exercises.

Another difference between traditional lunges and the T-Tapp Lunge Sequence is that you do not have to lunge as deep to be effective. Full fiber activation of your thigh muscles from knee to hip not only empowers your body to maximize muscle development, but also helps to stabilize and protect your knee.

Last of all, only one set of eight repetitions is all you need to trim, tone, and debulk your thighs. I know that is hard to believe when many of you have done high-repetition lunge programs, but you'll immediately feel the difference when you do the T-Tapp Lunge Sequence.

Start Position

It is important to establish correct body alignment before starting the side lunges. With your right foot pointing to the side and your left foot pointing to the front, make sure that the heel of your right foot is in alignment with the arch of your left foot. Your ankles should be in alignment with your shoulders, or if you are more flexible, widen your stance. Place your left hand below your waist and your right hand across your rib cage. Now slightly bend your right knee, push it out toward your little toe, and tuck your butt. Then twist your upper body without moving your lower body until your shoulders face forward. Now push your left thumb into your back and pull on your rib cage with your right hand to increase isometric activation of the muscles in your back and to stabilize your shoulders. You should feel deep activa-

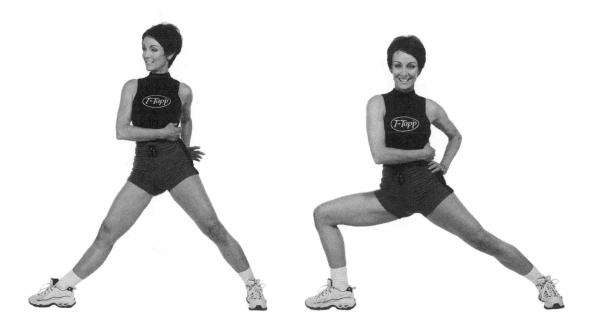

tion of the muscles along your spine. Then retighten your tuck and push your right knee out even more; you should feel deep activation of your upper right inner thigh (near groin) and stomach muscles. Last of all, try to maintain isometric activation of these muscles during the lunging leg movement. Now that your body is in correct alignment, let's lunge!

Step 1: Side Lunges

Keep pushing your knee out to KLT as you lunge into the side position (four counts). It is not necessary to lunge deep to receive results. In fact, in the beginning aim to achieve alignment between your right knee and ankle; never bend deeper than the end of your foot. It is more important to lunge with a shorter stance, less bend of knee, and with correct form than to lunge deep.

Form Check Keep your shoulders square to the front with your right knee in alignment with your right hip and shoulder. There should not be any weight on the ball of your right foot, and you should feel the arch of your foot lift inside your shoe.

Step 2

As you straighten your right leg, keep pushing your right knee out and tightening your tuck until your leg is straight (four counts).

Form Check Do not release your thigh muscles when your leg is straight, unless you want a bigger thigh. I usually say "tuck, twist, and tighten at the top" when training others to remind them to add a little turnout from their hip and knee when they tighten their tuck and thigh on count four.

TIP FOR BAD KNEES

If you have knee problems, tilt your upper body away while lunging and concentrate to maintain a tucked butt and a KLT position at all times.

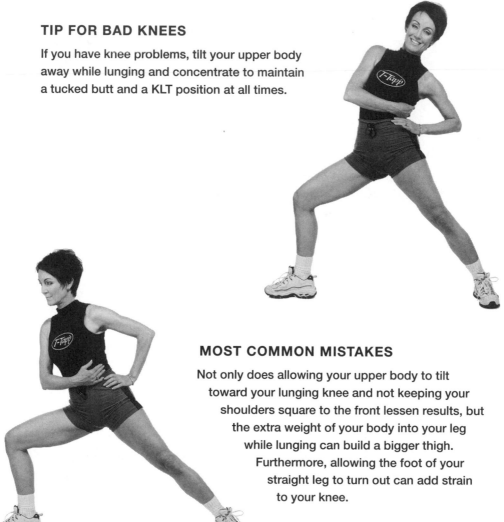

MOST COMMON MISTAKES

Not only does allowing your upper body to tilt toward your lunging knee and not keeping your shoulders square to the front lessen results, but the extra weight of your body into your leg while lunging can build a bigger thigh. Furthermore, allowing the foot of your straight leg to turn out can add strain to your knee.

As you can see from the photo, my image on the left demonstrates correct linear alignment between my shoulder, hip, knee, and ankle while in side lunge position. My image on the right, however, shows incorrect shoulder position (lat muscle attachment is not activated) and incorrect knee position (my knee is aiming to my big toe instead of my little toe).

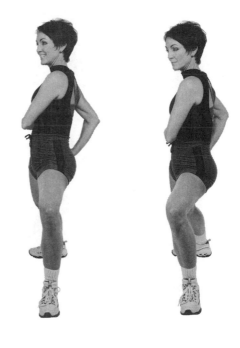

Repeat for a total of eight repetitions, eight counts each. Count each repetition as follows: lunge down with right knee (counts one to three) and hold (count four), then straighten right leg (counts five to seven) and hold with tuck/twist/tighten (count eight).

To prepare for front lunges, with same leg and without stopping, turn your upper body to the right and put the weight of your body into your right knee while you maintain KLT position. Lift your left heel and reset your left foot position to be straight (do not turn out as shown in the right image).

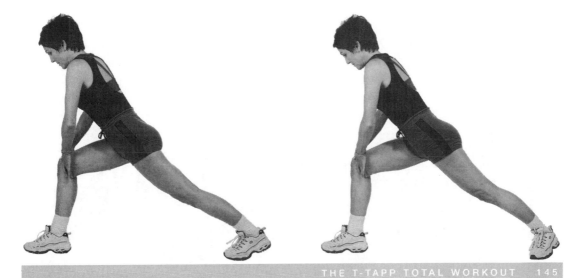

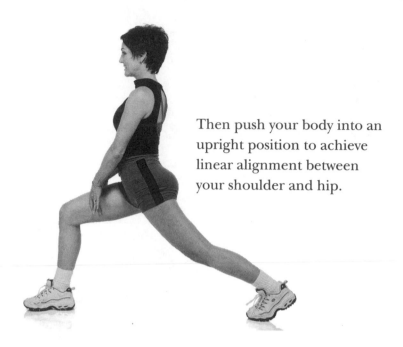

Then push your body into an upright position to achieve linear alignment between your shoulder and hip.

Step 3: Front Lunges

Bring your hands up in alignment with your elbows with palms up and thumbs back. Now push your elbows forward and pull your hands back. You should feel your upper back muscles activate. Your butt should be tucked as well, to maintain activation of your lower back and abdominal muscles. Now tuck your butt harder as you lift your left heel as high as you can while pressing your toes into the floor (two counts).

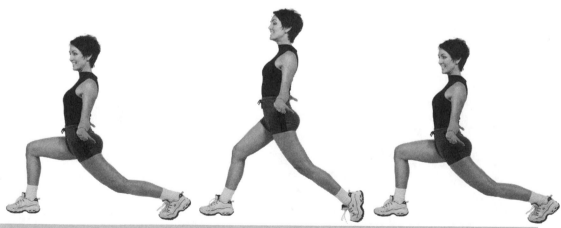

Form Check Keep your hips level with right knee pushing out and your left heel in alignment with your toes (no turnout). While pressing your toes into the floor, focus on keeping your weight equally distributed between your big and little toes. Your right knee should be slightly bent and in KLT on count two, but your left leg should be as straight as possible.

Step 4

Keep your left leg as straight as possible with toes forward while you lower your left heel (two counts). Your right knee should be in KLT position and in alignment with your right ankle. Your upper body should remain in an upright position with shoulders, elbows, hands, and hips in alignment.

Form Check Do not lunge forward. Your body should move straight up and down. The majority of your muscle fatigue should be in the front and top of your left thigh.

Repeat for a total of eight repetitions, four counts each. Count each front lunge as follows: tuck butt and lift left heel up (counts one and two), then push your right knee out as you lower your left heel (counts three and four).

Step 5

Push all of your body weight into your right leg, keeping the right knee out in KLT, as you pull your left leg back up even with your right leg. Then place your hands on both of your bent knees with thumbs on the inside and fingers on the outside. The weight of your upper body should be pressing equally into your knees to support your spine and give it a brief moment of rest after sustaining all those isometric contractions. Inhale big and exhale bigger (four counts).

Step 6

Then push your weight against your knees while you tuck your butt and chin until your arms straighten (counts one to four). Inhale big and exhale bigger to further stretch your spine and rib cage (counts five to eight). Then flip your palms and roll up, one vertebra at a time, until your body is in an upright position.

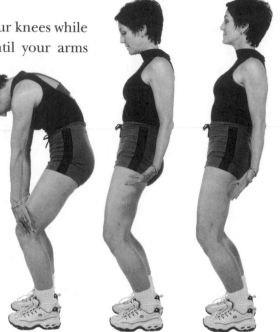

To prepare for drop lunges, step back with your left leg, keeping toes forward, shoulders back, and your right knee slightly bent and in KLT position.

Form Check Adjust your stance so that your left shoulder, hip, and knee are in perfect alignment. The object is not how far you can go down in the lunge but rather how well you keep your alignment.

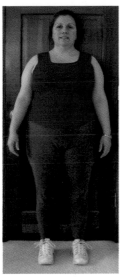 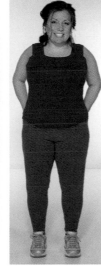

Debra Shafer proves that T-Tapp works fast and keeps on working. Check out her progress on page 21 at fourteen, sixty, and ninety days.

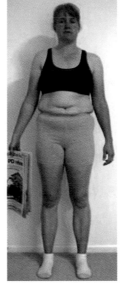 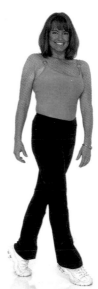

The incredible shrinking woman: Bekki Johnson not only dropped pregnancy pounds but said bye-bye to back fat as well!

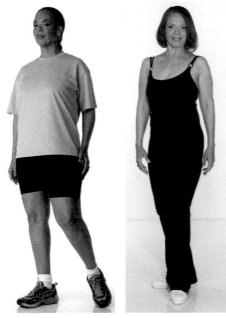

From walker to wow! After two back surgeries, Pat Richter not only looks better today than she did twenty years ago, she's now walking without pain—and no longer needs a walker.

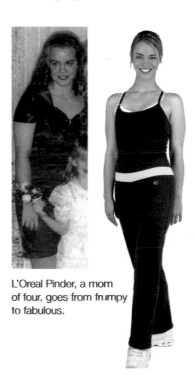

L'Oreal Pinder, a mom of four, goes from frumpy to fabulous.

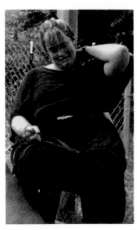

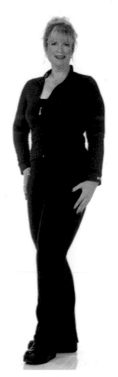

Check out Diane Stone's transformation from harried executive to hot mama!

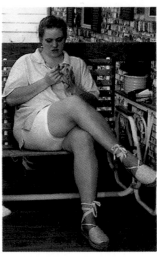

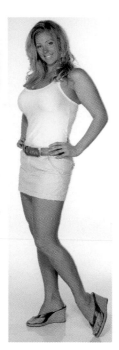

Heather Petrie calls her success a true Cinderella story: "I have a better body inside and out."

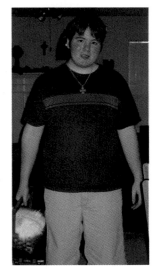

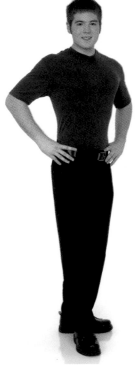

T-Tapp helped Chris Flores get his first date—"and she asked me!"

Sixty days . . .
and Julyn Harrison
has only just
begun.

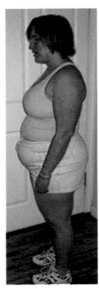 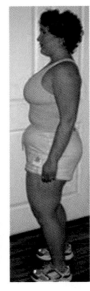 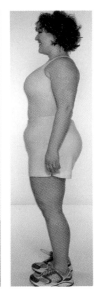

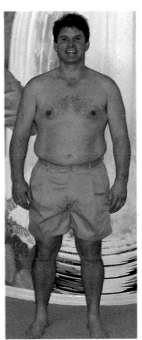 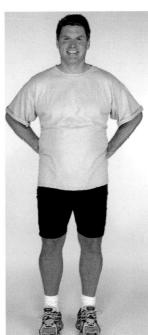

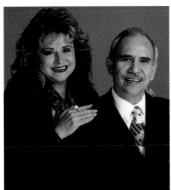

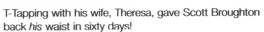
T-Tapping with his wife, Theresa, gave Scott Broughton
back *his* waist in sixty days!

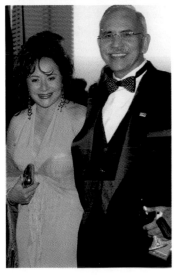

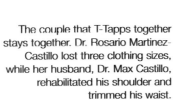

The couple that T-Tapps together
stays together. Dr. Rosario Martinez-
Castillo lost three clothing sizes,
while her husband, Dr. Max Castillo,
rehabilitated his shoulder and
trimmed his waist.

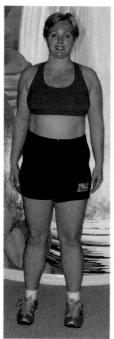 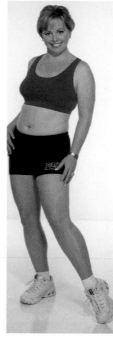

Lose inches after a hysterectomy? Theresa Broughton proves it's possible with T-Tapp. She lost 10.75 inches in two weeks!

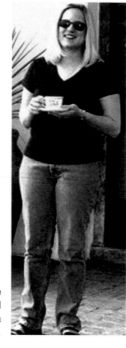 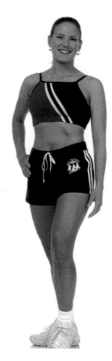

Nutritionists like Jenny Russell give T-Tapp a big thumbs-up.

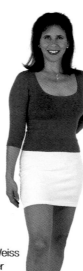

After T-Tapping, Margie Weiss became a magazine cover girl at age fifty!

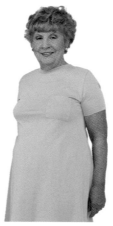 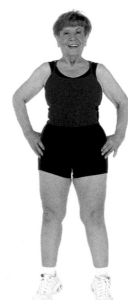

Seventy-eight-years-young Berei Brandenstein has turned back the clock with T-Tapp.

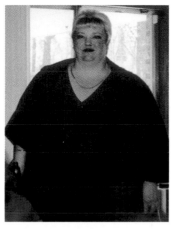

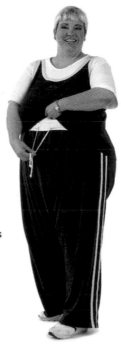

Bobbie Tribble says, "I lost six inches off my waist in two weeks just doing fifteen minutes of T-Tapp a day!"

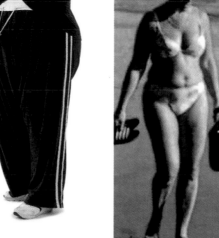

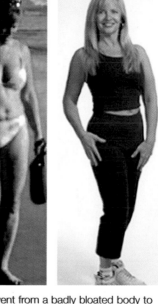

Sue Fetzner went from a badly bloated body to fit and firm.

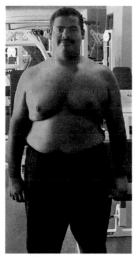

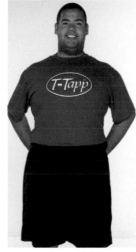

Paul Collier went from a couch potato to an active youth worker at his church.

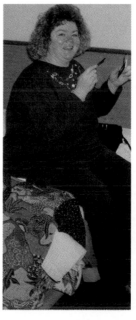

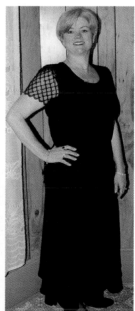

After two breast cancer surgeries in 2003, T-Tapper Deborah Baker felt "doomed." Now she's healthy, in shape, and inspiring others.

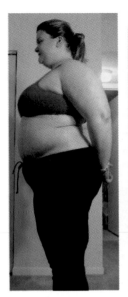 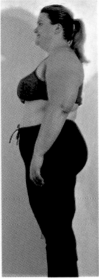

"I've developed what's known as the 'T-Tapp Glow,'" marvels law student Ally Hoagland, who lost fifty-three inches in sixty days—and counting.

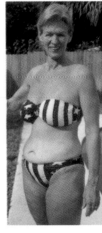 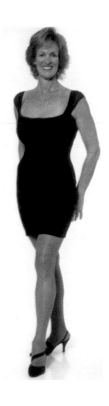

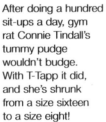

After doing a hundred sit-ups a day, gym rat Connie Tindall's tummy pudge wouldn't budge. With T-Tapp it did, and she's shrunk from a size sixteen to a size eight!

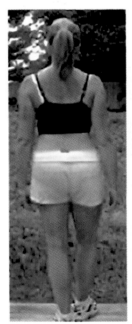 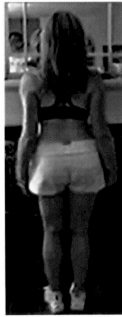

T-Tapp helped Shannon Keefe build a better butt in sixty days.

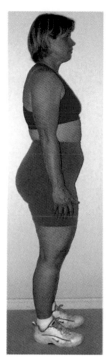
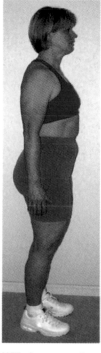

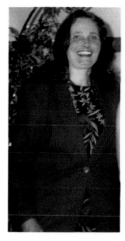
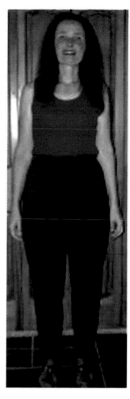

Not only did Donna McWillie lose more than twenty-one inches and eleven pounds in sixty days, but her carpal tunnel syndrome pain vanished. "I guess I've got that neuro-kinetic flow thing going on!"

Diagnosed with massive osteoporosis, Sylvia Hoffman could barely bend over to tie her shoes . . . but "T-Tapp has helped my back, knees, and energy level. And I look good for the first time in a long time!"

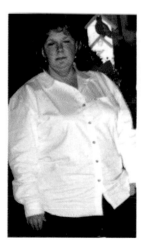
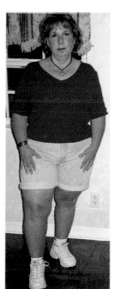

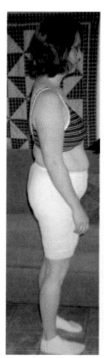
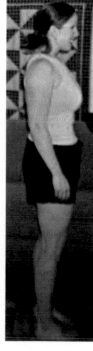

With T-Tapp, Sharlyn Bertrand has broken her twenty-year "fat cycle" forever.

In sixty days, Janice Metcalf flattened her tummy and perked her pecs!

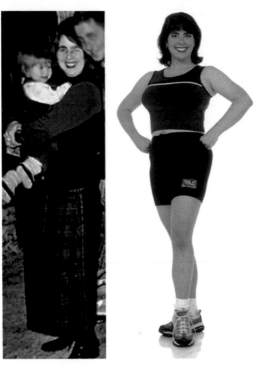

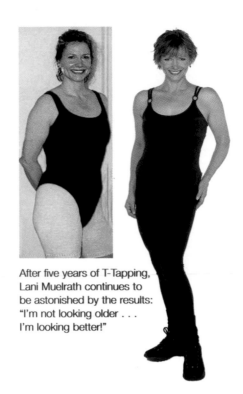

After five years of T-Tapping, Lani Muelrath continues to be astonished by the results: "I'm not looking older . . . I'm looking better!"

Labor and delivery were a piece of cake for T-Tapper Jeni Huffstedtler, who dropped her pregnancy weight in record time.

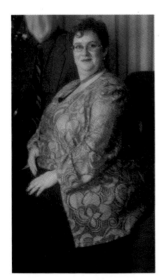

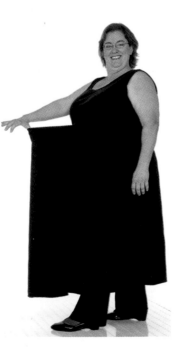

At eighty years young, T-Tapper Dorothy Trahan could be a swimsuit model! Va-va-va-voom!

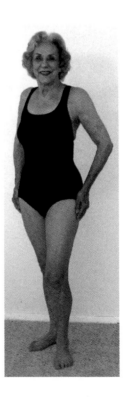

Having lost sixty inches and five pants sizes, Terri DeVillez credits T-Tapp with sending her energy level through the roof.

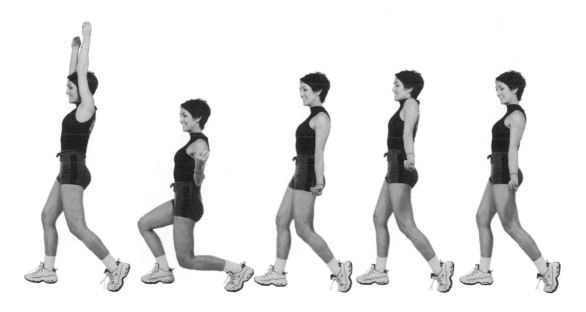

Step 7: Drop Lunges

Tuck your butt as you reach above your head (count one). Your arms should be in alignment with your ears, your elbows straight, and your fingertips pressing into your thumbs to create a doughnut hand position.

Step 8

Pull your arms down into a big W position with elbows forward and hands back in alignment with your shoulders as you lower your body and drop your left heel. Hold this position (four counts). Remain in same position but lift your heel and hold (four counts).

Form Check It is not important how low you are able to drop. Focus instead on keeping your shoulders, hips, and knees in linear alignment with butt tucked and shoulders back. Additionally, your right knee should always be pushing out into KLT position.

Step 9

Then continue to tuck and lift your left heel as high as you can while lifting your body and uncurling your arms from the W position with hands in doughnut position, palms facing up (counts one to four). Do not straighten your right leg; maintain a slight bend with a turnout position to KLT.

Form Check Concentrate on keeping your shoulders, elbows, hips, and knees in linear alignment. Always tuck your butt and push your right knee out more when coming up against gravity.

MOST COMMON MISTAKES

Standing with your feet too close (as shown in photo) or too wide will cause your left knee to be out of alignment from your hips and shoulders. This can create imbalance of muscle development and/or strain your right knee. Another common mistake is allowing your shoulders to drop forward as you lower your body or allowing them to roll forward when doing shoulder rolls. *Tip:* Tighten the muscles between your shoulder blades to help keep your shoulders back. Keeping shoulders back in alignment with your hips will maximize your body's ability to lose inches.

Step 10

Finish with one shoulder roll up and back. Repeat for a total of eight repetitions. Count each drop lunge as follows: reach (count one), pull and drop down into W position (counts two to four), lift heel (counts five to eight), then tuck and lift your body up (counts one to four) and finish with a shoulder roll (counts five to eight).

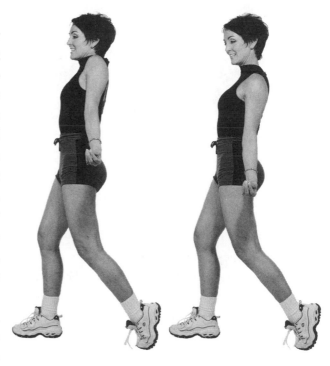

On counts seven and eight of your final drop lunge repetition, cross your arms in front of your chest with knees pushing out as you move your body to the left to face forward to the front. Continue to bring your arms down in front of your chest and extend them on out to the sides of your body. At the same time you move your arms, bend your knees deeper and push out into a full plié squat position.

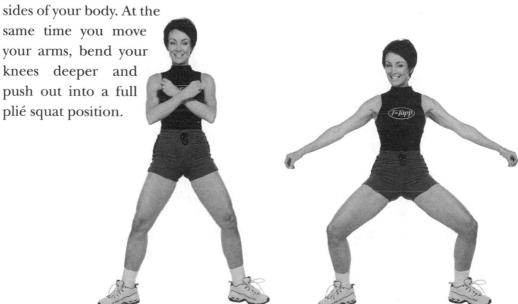

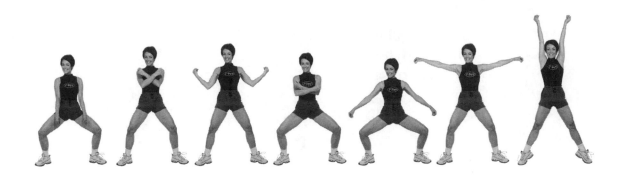

Step 11

Bring your arms down to the center of your body, cross them in front of your chest, and continue moving them until your hands are in a big W position (counts one and two). Your knees should be softly bent and in KLT position.

Form Check Keep your shoulders back while crossing arms in front (use those lats). Push your elbows forward and pull your hands back in alignment with your shoulders while in the W position. Then pull your elbows down until your hands are level with your shoulders.

Cross your arms back down in front of your chest as you lower your body into a full squat position. Continue moving your hands until your arms are out to your sides and in alignment with your shoulders. Keep your elbows straight as your arms continue to move up until they are in alignment with your ears (counts three and four). At the same time as your arms are reaching away and up, straighten your legs and lift your heels (counts five to eight).

Form Check Doughnut hands should face in toward your shoulders at the W position and when your arms are straight up (flip palms up when extended arms are level with your ears). Don't forget to tighten your butt tuck when your hands are above your head. Repeat for a total of four pliés.

Step 12

Finish drop lunges with one final W lat pull. Then kick each foot and lift each knee to release any muscle tension and to activate your lymphatic system to release excess lactic acid. Repeat. Then without stopping, put your body into the side lunge starting position with your left leg pointing to the side.

Repeat the entire Lunge Sequence (side-front-drop) with the left leg, Steps 1 to 12.

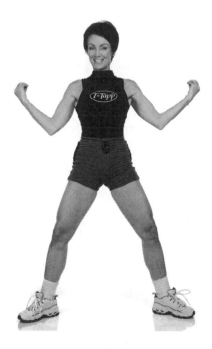

Then take a water break and proceed to Balance Sequence. Note: For those who have a higher level of fitness and/or desire more core challenge, proceed to Balance Sequence without stopping.

BALANCE SEQUENCE

The T-Tapp Balance Sequence is designed to focus on developing core muscle density, as well as to help strengthen joint muscle attachments on your hips, knees, and ankles. It involves simultaneous left-brain/right-brain movement, so it can be a bit challenging at first, but the movements work well to quickly improve neurokinetic connections for better body awareness and body balance.

Balance Sequence can be challenging, depending on various factors, but please do this movement without holding on to anything. Yes, you will lose your balance and touch the floor, but that's okay. Bobbling is good. In fact, as your body tries to center itself, it is activating muscle attachments along your spine—which is the secret to developing core muscles with density.

Balance Sequence can be done as a stand-alone exercise if you need to improve your coordination and ability to balance without fatigue factors, but for optimal results and cardiac conditioning, you should do it immediately after the T-Tapp Lunge Sequence.

Start Position

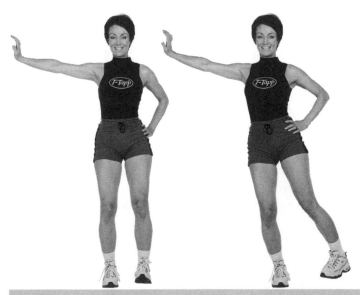

For optimal results, it is important to establish correct body alignment and foot position before starting the side leg lifts. Extend your right hand level with your shoulders, keeping your elbows straight and knuckles pulled back. Your left hand should be below your waist with your thumb pushing in to help pull your left shoulder back and stabilize it with better isometric contraction (leverage isometrics). Now bend your right knee, tuck your butt, push your right knee out, and shift your weight into your right leg. Then pull up the toes of your left foot while you press your left heel down and let your body establish some balance. Keep your left knee slightly bent so you can turn out your left knee and aim it to your little toe on your left foot. Now turn your left foot in, but keep it flexed, with your heel pressing down and your toes pulling up. Remember, bobbling is good. Now you're ready to begin.

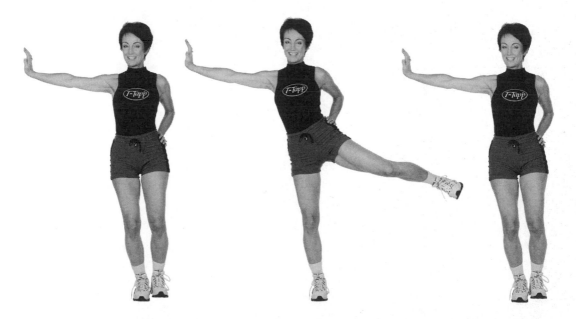

Step 1: Side Leg Lift

Tuck your butt and push your right knee out as you lift your left leg with toes forward (count one). The height of your leg lift is not as important as keeping your butt tucked and toes forward.

Form Check Although your toes may face forward at the top of your leg lift, always begin each lift with your toes turned in. *Tip:* The combination of pressing your heel down and pulling your toes up will help you stabilize your ankle and foot position during the lift.

Now pull your shoulders back and tighten the muscles between your shoulder blades to help stabilize the position of your shoulder. You should also feel your latissimus dorsi muscles activate along the sides of your back. Shoulder and hip alignment during leg movement is very important for core muscle development and to flatten your tummy. In fact, you should feel your core muscles activate with every leg lift.

Step 2

Then tighten your tummy as you lower your left leg all the way down (counts two to four). Keep your heel-down/toe-up position at all times and do not touch the floor.

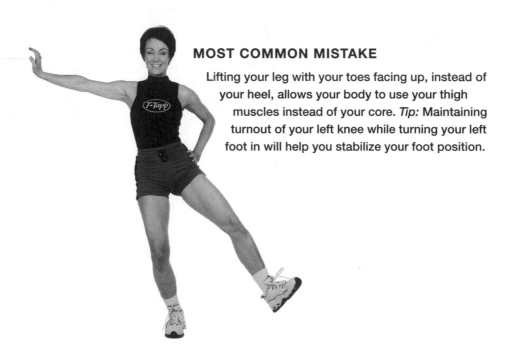

MOST COMMON MISTAKE

Lifting your leg with your toes facing up, instead of your heel, allows your body to use your thigh muscles instead of your core. *Tip:* Maintaining turnout of your left knee while turning your left foot in will help you stabilize your foot position.

Repeat for a total of eight repetitions, four counts each. Count each side leg lift repetition as follows: tuck as you lift leg up quick (count one), then tighten and tuck as you lower leg down slow (counts two to four). Proceed to combo leg lifts without stopping.

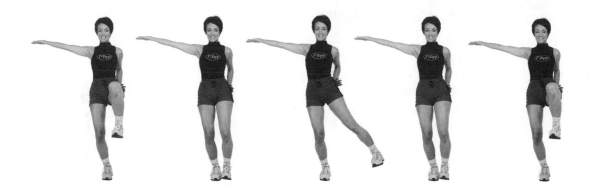

Step 3: Combo Leg Balance

Flip your right palm up, pull your left elbow back, and tuck your butt while you lift your left knee up level with your hips or waist. Hold this position while you check your form and allow your body to establish better balance before doing the combo leg lifts. Remember, bobbling is good. Inhale, exhale, and check your form within four counts.

Form Check Your right knee should be bent in KLT position. Your shoulders should be back in alignment with your hips. Your left knee should be in alignment with your left shoulder, and your left ankle should be in alignment with your left knee. Your left foot should be flexed and pointing forward with toes up and heel down. Form is important for optimal results and core muscle development. Now you're ready to begin.

Step 4: Combo Leg Lifts

Press your left heel down as you extend your left leg nearly straight and without touching the floor (count one). Then tighten your tuck and push your right knee out while you do a lateral side leg lift with toes up and slightly turned in (count two). Lower your left leg back to center position without releasing form or touching the floor (count three). Then tuck your butt and tighten your tummy as you lift your left knee back up (count four).

MOST COMMON MISTAKES

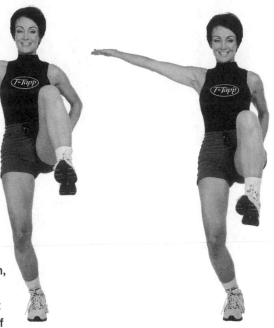

Not maintaining correct alignment between your knee and shoulder and between your ankle and knee are the most common mistakes when doing combo leg lifts. Even though my image on the left shows an advanced level of lift and correct alignment on the right side of my body, my left knee is aiming to the inside of my left shoulder and my ankle is out of alignment. Even though I'm only slightly out of alignment, it still releases activation of my transverse abdominus muscle in my lower abdomen, as well as my thigh muscles where they attach on my hip joint. Unfortunately, not only does this lessen the effectiveness of my knee lift, it can also add inches to my outer thigh, where saddlebag fat likes to settle! Remember, active muscle movement burns fat for fuel, and proper form empowers your muscles to work harder. Now compare images. My image on the right still shows an advanced level of lift, but having my right palm up, left elbow back, and right knee pushed out even more helps improve and stabilize the position of my left knee. *Note:* It is okay to alternate hand positions during side leg lifts with palms up or palms facing to the side with your wrist pushing out and your knuckles pulling back.

Lifting your knee to the outside of your shoulder with your foot aiming to the center of your body is another common mistake that creates inactivation of your lower abdominal and inner thigh muscles. Linear alignment from knee to ankle is important for core muscle development.

Repeat for a total of eight repetitions, four counts each. Proceed to next move (back leg lifts with flex foot) without touching your foot to the floor.

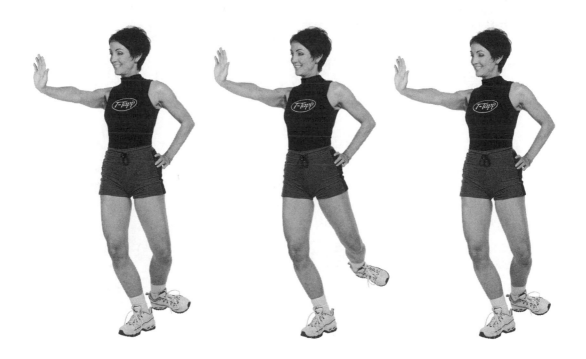

Step 5: Back Leg Lifts with Flex Foot

Place your left foot in flexed position behind your right leg with heel down, toes up, and the arch of your left foot in alignment with your right heel. At the same time you move your left leg back, bring your right arm forward with the knuckles of your hand and your shoulder pulling back. Then tuck your butt and turn your left knee out as far as you can for an optimal T position with toes pointing to the side. Keep both your shoulders back in alignment with your hips and your butt tucked at all times. *Tip for beginners:* Place your feet on the floor in a T position, with the heel of your right foot perpendicular to the instep of your left foot. Inhale big and exhale bigger to give your body a moment of rest. Then shift the weight of your body into your right leg, lift left foot off the floor, and establish your balance while putting your body into correct position with correct form.

Step 6

Now lift your left leg straight back (count one) and lower it until the arch of your left foot touches your right heel (count two). Do not touch the floor.

MOST COMMON MISTAKE

Allowing your upper body to tilt forward releases activation of your lower back and abdominal muscles, and not keeping your foot turned out to best ability (T position) releases abdominal, thigh, and hip muscles.

Repeat Step 6 for a total of eight repetitions, two counts each.

Step 7

Continue lifting your leg, but this time point your foot as you lift (count one) and flex as you touch your heel (count two). Do not touch the floor, and maintain form to the best of your ability. Repeat Step 7 for a total of eight repetitions, two counts each.

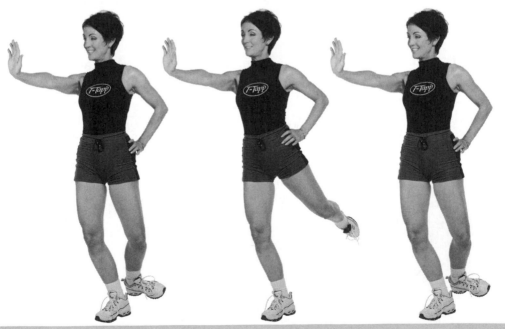

Step 8

At the end of the eighth repetition of back leg lifts with point and flex, pull your left knee up to the front of your body with toes forward, heel down and in alignment. At the same time, your right arm moves out to your side in alignment with your right shoulder and with palm facing down (counts one and two). Then bring your left arm to the front of your body in alignment with your left shoulder with palm facing down (counts three and four). Inhale (counts five and six) and during the exhale (counts seven and eight) pull your shoulders back.

Step 9

Point your toes as you swing your left leg back (counts one and two). At the same time you swing-kick, your arms reach away, but keep your shoulder muscles tight. Keep your butt tucked with right knee bent in KLT position at all times.

Form Check Focus not on how high you can swing-kick, but instead you should focus on how high you can swing-kick without release of form.

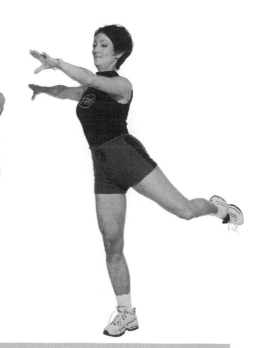

Then pull your shoulders back without bending your elbows and tuck your butt as you swing your left knee back to starting position with a flat foot (counts three and four). Repeat Step 9 for a total of eight repetitions, two counts each. Proceed to Step 10, front lat presses, without stopping.

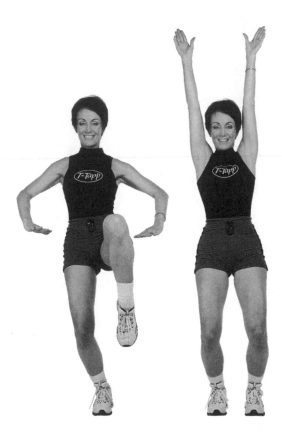

Step 10: Front Lat Presses

After completing the last repetition of swing-kicks, press your hands down to below your hips with fingers turned in. At the same time, bring your left knee up with a pointed foot, keeping your knee and ankle in alignment with your left shoulder (counts one and two). Then place your left foot on the floor at the same time you reach with your hands above your head until your elbows are straight and in alignment with your ears (counts three and four). Repeat the front lat press, lifting your right knee up (counts one and two) and reaching with your hands up (counts three and four).

Form Check Pull your shoulders back and push your chest forward to maximize activation of your lats every time you lift your knee. Tuck your butt and push your knees out every time you reach above your head.

MOST COMMON MISTAKE

The left image shows incorrect knee/ankle alignment along with incorrect hand position; both of these common mistakes inactivate core muscles and lessen results. Your hands should be out to the sides of your body and below your hips. The right image shows the same mistakes, but the side view allows you to better see how my upper body is tilting forward with my shoulders in front of my hips. Those who have weak abdominal muscles and/or weak upper back muscles tend to use the momentum of their upper body pulling forward to help pull their knee up.

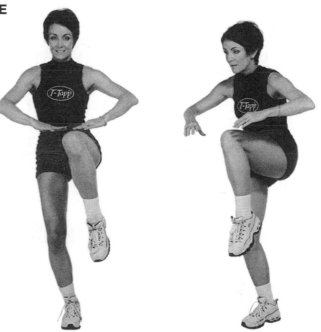

Repeat Step 10 for a total of eight repetitions, four counts each. Proceed to Step 11, puppet pulls, without stopping.

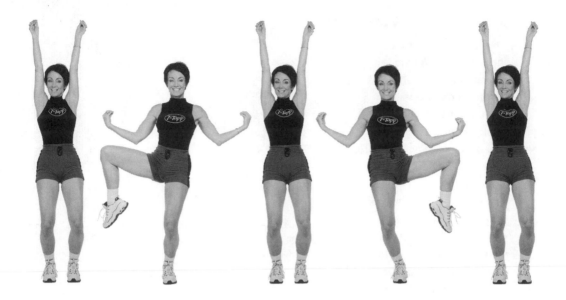

Step 11: Puppet Pulls

Reach above your head with your hands in doughnut position and your elbows straight in alignment with your ears. Keep your butt tucked and knees out into KLT position (counts one and two). Then pull your arms down until your hands create a big W and are level with your shoulders (counts three and four). At the same time you pull your hands down, lift your right knee, with toes pointed, out to the right side in alignment with your right shoulder and/or behind your right ear. As you lower your right leg with toes forward and knees out in KLT, reach up again until your elbows are straight (counts five and six). Then pull your arms down into a W while lifting your left knee out (counts seven and eight).

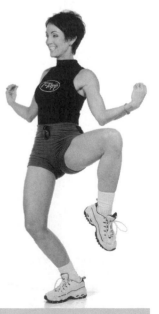

Form Check Your ankles, knees, elbows, and hands should be in alignment with your shoulders as shown in photo. Additionally, be sure to twist your wrist (doughnut hand) each time your pull your hands down (palms face in) and every time you reach up (palms face forward).

MOST COMMON MISTAKE

Allowing your elbows to pull back causes your shoulders to pronate forward, thus creating more trapezius and biceps muscle activation in comparison to your latissimus dorsi muscle. Allowing your knee to ankle to lose alignment inactivates your abdominal, hip, and thigh muscles. Linear alignment is very important for optimal core muscle development. Always strive to achieve correct linear alignment to the best of your ability and you *will* achieve results, even if you are not able to create exact duplication of my body position.

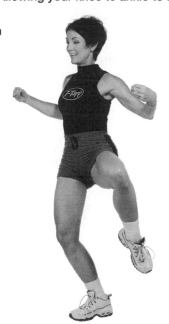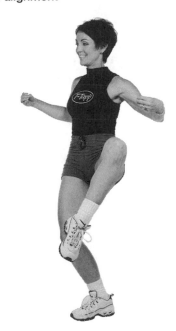

Repeat Step 11 for a total of eight repetitions, eight counts each.

Now repeat entire Balance Sequence from the beginning (Steps 1 to 11), lifting with your right leg. You can take a water break first, if needed.

AIRPLANES

The sequential movements in Airplanes are designed to progressively stretch all of the muscles in your core and assist your body's lymphatic function as well as strengthen and increase flexibility of your shoulders, hips, knees, and spine. Furthermore, the combination of deep breathing while twisting your spine with lower body KLT positioning maximizes lymphatic flow. Additionally, maintaining linear alignment while moving your torso in a horizontal plane strengthens your abdominal and back muscles due to the extra gravitational pull. Best of all, your metabolic processing gets an extra boost during Airplanes for optimal fat burning. Feel the heat!

Step 1: Airplane Stretch

For optimal results, it is important to establish correct body alignment before stretching your spine. Assume a flat back position with your shoulders level to your hips and arch your butt up to comprehensively

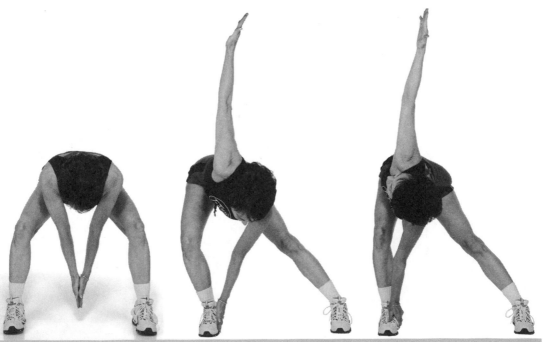

activate your back, abdominal, and thigh muscles. Your feet should be at least shoulder width apart with toes facing forward and knees pushing out in alignment with your ankles. Now shift your weight over to the right until your right knee is lunging past your little toe. Make sure your shoulders and hips are still in alignment. Then place your left hand on the inside of your left foot and your right hand above your head in alignment with your right shoulder. Your right thumb should be facing forward and your palm should be facing out to the right.

Once your body is in correct body alignment, turn your head and look up at your right hand. Inhale big and exhale bigger (four counts). You should feel your rib cage expand and all your torso muscles stretch when you inhale and you should feel the muscles between your ribs pull them closer together and all your torso muscles cinch in while you exhale. Repeat.

Then keep your shoulders in alignment with your hips while you shift your weight over to the left. Establish correct form before you look up. Repeat inhale and exhale twice (four counts each).

Repeat Step 1, but increase the intensity of your stretch by lunging deeper, as well as inhaling and exhaling bigger (eight counts) for a total of two each side.

Step 2: Transition to Lateral Movement

Return your body to center and lower your hips into a squat position with toes forward. As you lower your body, push your elbows into your knees and keep your shoulders back. Your knees should be in alignment with your ankles or on the outside of your little toes if you are flexible. Keep pushing your knees out and hold this position for four counts. Then lift your upper body back into a level position and place your palms together with elbows straight. Now pull your shoul-

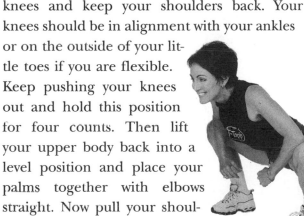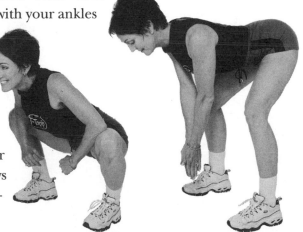

ders back, arch your butt up, and keep your knees out as you prepare to move in lateral alignment from right to left.

MOST COMMON MISTAKES

These two images show the two most common errors that occur when doing Airplanes: feet too far apart and shoulders lower than hips. Linear alignment is important for comprehensive activation of your muscles. Having too wide a stance not only lessens results in your thighs and stomach, it also creates an imbalance of muscle activation at your knee and can cause knee strain. It is better to have a shorter stance than one that's too wide. Increase the width of your stance only to the point where you can maintain knee to ankle alignment.

Furthermore, when your shoulders become lower than your hips, your back and abdominal muscles will not able to maintain comprehensive activation. Linear alignment empowers your muscles to move with resistance without adding weight. However, subconsciously your body will seek to move in the path of least resistance, especially when tired. So whenever you feel like your muscles are getting tired, check your T-Tapp form—especially linear alignment.

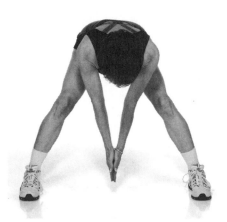 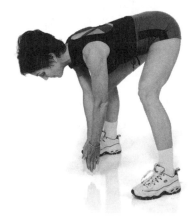

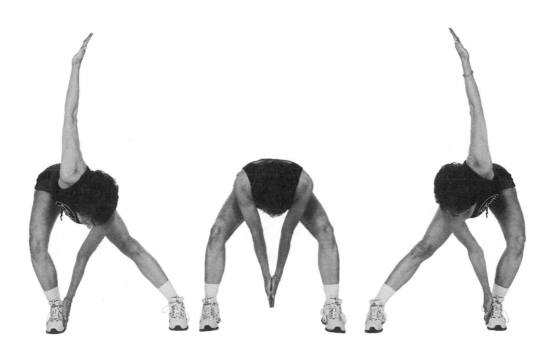

Step 3: Airplane Movement

Continue moving laterally, alternating from right to left as shown in the photos, with a clap in the middle. Keep your spine centered with your face looking at the floor.

Form Check Be sure to bend your knees deep enough. Aim for your little toe, or a little further if you are more flexible.

MOST COMMON MISTAKE

Hyperextending your arm behind your back not only lessens results, it can create strain to your shoulder. Your wrist should be in alignment with your shoulder.

Repeat for a total of eight repetitions, four counts each. Count each Airplane as follows: flat back lunge to right with right arm up (count one), then clap (count two) as you move through center, continue flat back lunge to left with left arm up (count three), then clap (count four) as you move through center.

Step 4: Transition Stretch

Return your body to center position. Place your elbows on your knees and shift all of your body weight there. Then lower your butt as far as you can. As you lower your butt, push your knees out with your elbows to achieve optimal hamstring and inner thigh stretch, as well as lymphatic drainage. Inhale, exhale, and hold this position for four counts.

Form Check Your knees should be in alignment with your ankles, or on the outside of your little toes if you are more flexible.

Then bring your heels in without moving any other part of your body (count one). As you bring your toes forward, lift your butt (count two). Then bring your heels inward (count three) and finish with your toes forward (count four).

Form Check It is not necessary to have your hips and shoulders level as you walk your feet back into T-Tapp stance.

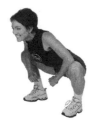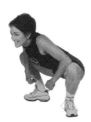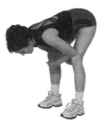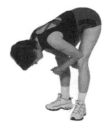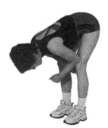

Step 5

Place your hands on the outside of your calves with elbows out and head relaxed. Inhale big and exhale bigger. This stretch should feel really good on your lower back.

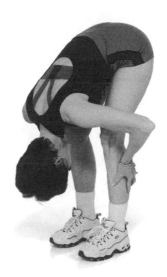

Step 6: Head Rocks

Push your knees out while pushing your hands in (leverage isometrics for your back). Then tighten your butt to activate a deeper stretch within your gluteal and hamstring muscles. All of your muscles should be tight, with comprehensive isometric activation for spinal support, except your head and neck. Relax your muscles from your neck up and gently rock your head four times.

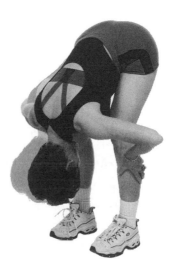

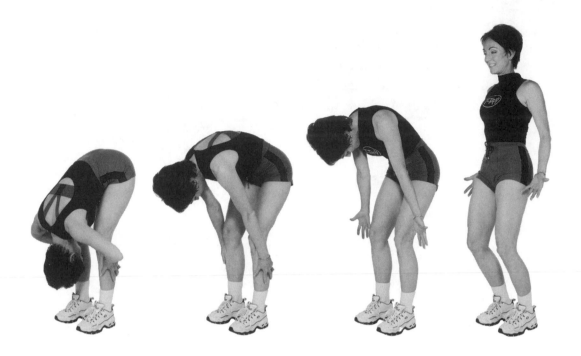

Step 7: Spinal Roll-Up

Tuck your butt and curl your back until your arms are straight and you feel a tug in your lower back. Once you feel this tug, tuck your butt harder and pull without releasing your hands for a total of four counts (count one to four). Then flip your palms forward with thumbs out to the sides and reach down as you continue to roll up one vertebra at a time until you are in an upright position (counts five to eight). Finish your spinal roll-up with one big shoulder roll up (counts one and two) and back (counts three and four).

Now take a water break before proceeding to Thread the Needle.

THREAD THE NEEDLE

Many consider Thread the Needle the T-Tapp move that reveals the most in regard to left-brain/right-brain coordination, core density, and body balance. It challenges all fitness levels and will continue to challenge even as you become stronger. I created Thread the Needle to provide body sculpting from your waist to your knees, as well as to develop core density all the way up along your spine. Core and spinal strength, as well as flexibility of your hip joints, will improve with time, so always go to your personal max, and eventually you'll be able to do this mind/body movement without touching the floor. Remember, bobbling is good, so do not hold on to anything. Just keep your upper back muscles tight with shoulders back and butt tucked with knee out to stabilize your spine. Then tuck and tighten as you move, and feel your muscles maximize, layer by layer, from the inside out!

Step 1: U-Swing Setup

Assume a slight lunge position with your left knee bent and pushing out to KLT, butt tucked and shoulders back. Lift your shoulders as you inhale big (counts one and two). Then roll your shoulders back and down as you exhale bigger (counts three and four).

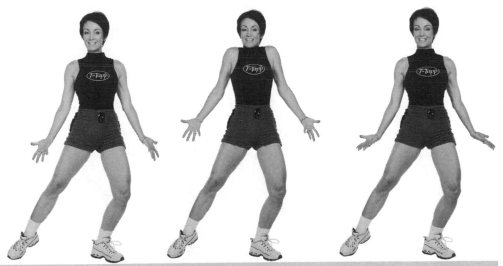

Form Check Twist your thumbs back while reaching down for optimal shoulder alignment and lat activation along with release of any muscle tension in your neck (trapezius).

Step 2: U-Swing Squats

While keeping your upper back tight, your butt tucked, and your left knee bent in KLT, use your right knee to create a big U-swing motion from left to right. Your shoulders should not move while you move your hands in opposition to your knees. Bring your right knee across your body over to your left (count one). Then swing your right knee down without touching the floor (count two) and back up over to your right side as high as you can (count three) and down into a full plié squat position with your butt tucked and knees out (count four). Then hold plié squat position for four counts with optimal form.

Form Check Keep your shoulders back in alignment with your hips and turn your right thumb back as far as you can to stabilize your right shoulder. During squat position, tuck your butt, pull your shoulders back, and push your knees out to your personal max.

Repeat for a total of four repetitions, eight counts each. Count each U-swing squat as follows: right knee over to your left with left hand on right side (count one), right knee down to center with both hands down (count two), right knee over to your right with right hand on left side (count three), right knee down on your right side in squat position with right hand still over on your left side (count four), hold squat position (counts five to eight).

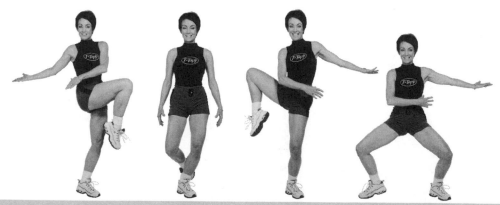

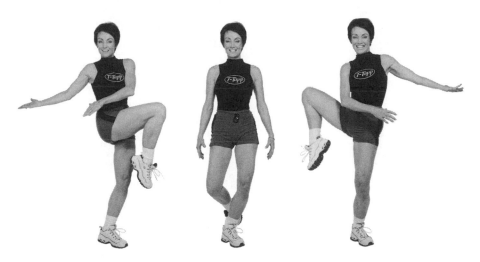

Step 3: U-Swings

Reset your body with another shoulder roll (Step 1) and start doing Step 2, but instead of ending in a squat position for the final count, keep moving your right knee back down (count four) and up over to your left (count one) without stopping or touching the floor. Continue moving your right knee in a U-swing pattern with your hands in opposition without touching the floor until final repetition. There is a bit of momentum while doing U-swings, but do not go too fast. To receive optimal results, focus on maintaining isolation of your upper body from your lower body with smooth equal speed.

Form Check Tuck and tighten your tummy every time you bring your knee up to maximize inch loss, and never, ever straighten your supportive knee. Keep your left knee bent and pushing out to your little toe at all times in KLT.

Repeat for a total of eight repetitions, four counts each. Count each U-swing as follows: right knee over to your left with left hand on right side (count one), right knee down to center with both hands down (count two), right knee over to your right with right hand on left side (count three), right knee down to center with both hands down (count four). Repeat. On the final repetition, drop your right knee down on your right side (no squat) and proceed to Step 4.

Step 4: Set Up for Cross/Cross–Back/Lifts

Extend your arms at shoulder height with palms facing down and place your right knee behind your left leg with toes touching the floor. Bend your left knee and push it out to KLT position. Tighten the muscles between your shoulder blades and inhale (counts one and two). Then during the exhale (counts three and four), reach out with your arms like someone is pulling your hands.

Form Check Reaching out enables greater isometric activation of all the muscles that attach to your shoulder, especially the lats.

Step 5: Cross/Cross–Back/Lifts

Lift your right knee up on the right side of your body with your toes pointed waist high and without moving your upper body (count one). Then without dropping your right knee lower than your waist, cross your right knee over to the left side of your body. At the same time, bend your left elbow and bring your left hand in front of your chest (count two). Then extend your left hand back out and bring your right knee back over to the right side of your body (count three). Then drop your right knee in turned-out position behind your left leg without touching the floor (count four). Without stopping, tuck your butt to

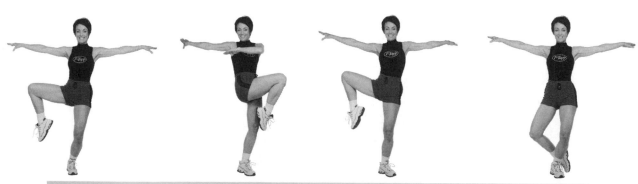

help you bring your right knee back up into the count one position and repeat the sequence eight times.

Form Check It is important to keep your lower body isolated at all times with your butt tucked and left knee pushing out, as well as your shoulders back and in alignment with your hips. Movement of your left elbow bending in and extending back out is done with a bit of momentum to help your body increase range of motion and flexibility of the muscles that attach at your hip (hip flexors). It is okay to slightly bend your left knee a little deeper when you drop your right knee behind your left leg, but never straighten your supportive knee. Keep your toes pointed at all times. Did you realize that pointing your toes increases the intensity of muscle activation within your abdominal muscles? Focus on pointing your toes to your personal max and feel the difference. Who ever thought that pointing toes could help flatten your tummy? Neurokinetic transmission is the secret to success.

Repeat for a total of eight repetitions, four counts each. Count each cross/cross–back/lift as follows: lift right knee up (count one), cross right knee to left (count two), cross right knee back to right (count three), and drop right knee down without touching floor (count four).

Step 6: Little Pliés

Assume a plié stance that is wide enough for your shoulders to be in alignment with your ankles or, if you are more flexible, in alignment to the inside of your heels (as shown in photo on p. 178). Place your hands slightly below your hips with your elbows aiming back, your thumbs pressing in, and your fingers pulling away. You should feel the muscles in your back tighten and your shoulders pull back into better alignment with your hips. Maintain this isometric leverage at all times. Now lower your body with your butt tucked and your knees pushing out (count one) and then, when coming up against gravity, tuck and push KLT even more until your legs are straight with your knees turned out (count two).

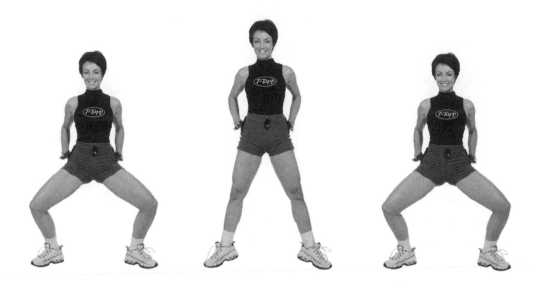

Form Check Do not relax your thighs or tuck when your legs are straight. Your feet should only be turned out at an angle of approximately 30 degrees. Too much turnout lessens results and can cause strain to your ankle and/or knee.

Repeat for a total of four repetitions, two counts each for a total of eight counts. Count each little plié as follows: bend knees and lower body down (count one), straighten knees and lift body up (count two).

Now repeat the entire sequence, Steps 1 to 6, using your right leg to support and your left leg to move. On count eight of Step 6, hold and proceed immediately to Step 7.

Step 7: Alternating Heel Lifts

Before starting, hold your plié position and focus on form. Your knees should be in alignment with your ankles or, if you are more flexible, in alignment with the end of your feet. Your shoulders should be back in alignment with your hips, your butt tucked, and your knees pushing out to KLT. Both your elbows and hands should be in alignment with your shoulders when you are seen from the side. Your palms should be facing up with thumbs back to the best of your ability and be in

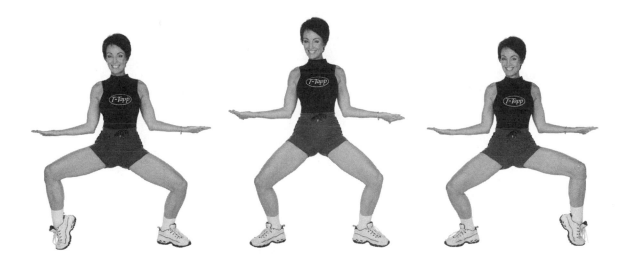

alignment with your elbows and shoulders. Now that every muscle in your body is activated and you're in linear alignment to the best of your ability, let's get started.

Lift your right heel as high as you can (count one), then lower right heel (count two), then lift your left heel as high as you can (count three), then lower your left heel (count four).

Form Check Keep pushing your elbows forward and pulling your hands back to maintain correct upper body position. Your elbows should be close to your body. Keep tucking your butt and pushing KLT to the best of your ability at all times while lifting heels.

Repeat for a total of four repetitions, four counts each. Count each alternating heel lift as follows: lift right heel (count one), lower right heel (count two), lift left heel (count three), and lower left heel (count four). Proceed to Step 8 without stopping.

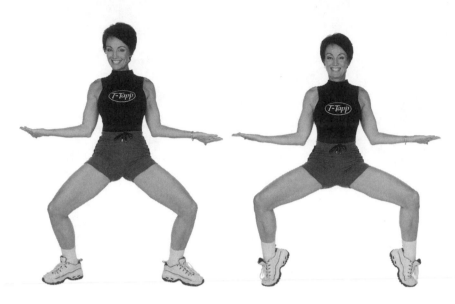

Step 8: Heel Lifts

While maintaining the same body position and form as detailed in Step 7, continue lifting your heels, but lift both at the same time. By now your muscles are probably getting tired, so really focus on form. In addition to all form details discussed in Step 7, also focus on not letting your ankles roll out. It is important to maintain correct ankle and heel alignment with your knees when lifting the weight of your body against gravity.

MOST COMMON MISTAKE

Allowing your upper body to tilt forward usually occurs when your back and abdominal muscles get tired. Even just a little tilt will alter results because it will cause your shoulders to come in front of your hips, and it doesn't take much movement forward to inactivate your lower back and abdominal muscles. Compare my correct image on the left to my incorrect image on the right and you can easily see how my elbows, wrists, and butt tuck have been altered as a result of my shoulders being in front of my hips.

Repeat for a total of four repetitions, two counts each. Count each heel lift as follows: lift heels (count one) and lower heels (count two). Repeat for a total of eight counts, then proceed to Step 9 without stopping.

Step 9: Finale

While you straighten your legs back up to a standing position (counts one to four) it is important to maintain isolation of your upper and lower body at all times. Keep tucking your butt and pushing your knees out for lower body isolation, and keep pushing your elbows forward and pulling your hands back for upper body isolation. Finish with one final "tuck, twist, and tighten" contraction when your legs are straight. You should feel major stretching and fatigue factors happening along the insides of your legs.

Form Check Your knees should be turned out even when your legs are straight.

Finish with two sets of alternating right/left little kicks and right/left knee lifts to help release muscle tension and lactic acid accumulation. It should feel good when you lift/touch and kick/kick.

Now take a water break and proceed to Runner's Stretch.

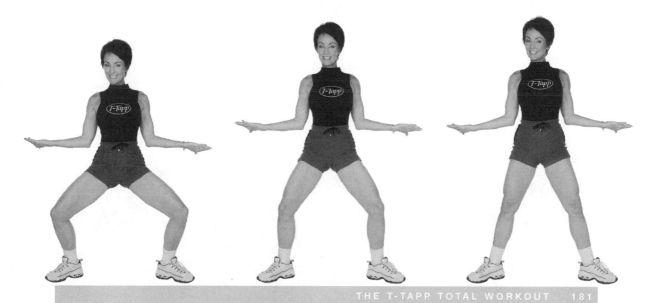

RUNNER'S STRETCH

Runner's Stretch is designed to stretch all of the muscles in your thighs, back, and butt and help your body eliminate any accumulation of lactic acid from muscle fatigue. If the buildup of lactic acid isn't eliminated, muscle soreness is much more pronounced due to inflammation of muscle tissue. This stretch also assists lymphatic flow and boosts metabolic function for optimal fat burning.

Remember, levels of flexibility vary from one person to the next but will improve with time and practice. During Runner's Stretch, your goal should be to stretch to your own personal max without compromising form.

Step 1: Lunges

Lunge forward with your right knee and extend your left leg back. Your left hip, knee, and ankle should be in alignment with toes forward, and your right knee should be in alignment with your right ankle, or to the end of your foot if you are more flexible. Never extend your knee past your toes or you can strain your knee. Your hands should be on either side of your right leg with thumbs facing inward and fingers pointing to side (not front) to establish correct shoulder position.

Form Check The palms of your hands should not be touching the floor. Your right knee should be pushing to your little toe (KLT), or a little further if you are more flexible. Hold this position for four counts.

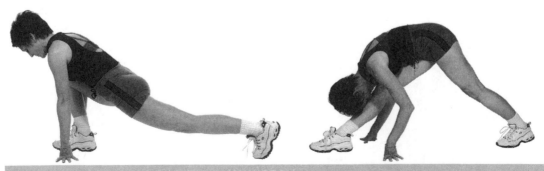

Keep your upper body in contact with your right thigh as you straighten your right knee as far as you can, keeping both shoulders square and your hips level. While holding this position for four counts, your head and neck should be relaxed, with both of your knees turned out into KLT.

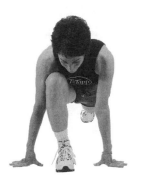
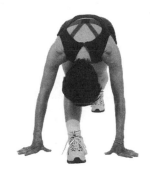

Form Check Keep your tummy tight and tighten the muscles between your shoulder blades to pull your shoulders back. Be sure to inhale and exhale during lunge and stretch.

MOST COMMON MISTAKE

Allowing your back foot to turn out releases activation of the muscles that attach to your left hip. Not only does this lessen the stretch within your left thigh, is also creates muscle imbalance in your hip and spine.

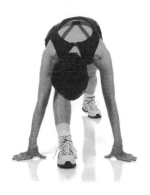

Repeat for a total of three repetitions. Count each lunge as follows: bend right knee and lunge (counts one to four), straighten right leg and stretch (counts five to eight). Continue to hold this position and begin Step 2 without stopping.

Step 2: Tighten/Release Stretch

While maintaining an extended stretch with your right knee straight, or to the best of your ability, tighten your thigh muscles and hold (counts one and two). Then let your right knee slightly bend and relax your thigh muscles (counts three and four). Repeat straighten/bend knee movement with your thigh muscles tightening and relaxing for a total of four times. Then straighten your right knee and proceed to Step 3 without stopping.

Form Check Keep your tummy muscles tight and your shoulders back to the best of your ability while tightening and relaxing your thigh. Recheck position of your left foot and make sure it is still straight without any turnout.

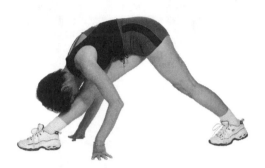 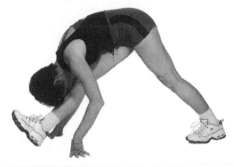

Step 3: Lift/Touch Toes

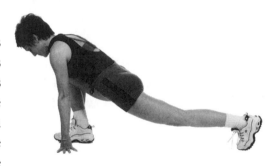

While keeping your right knee as straight as you can and your hips level, lift and touch your right toes up and down to the floor three times (counts one to three). Then bend your right knee and lunge (count four) and inhale and exhale while you hold this position (counts five to eight).

Step 4: Transition

Pull your left leg in toward your body (it should feel heavy) and bring your right foot back so that both of your feet are in alignment with toes forward. Rest for four counts and proceed to Step 5.

Step 5: Spine Roll-Up with Shoulder Roll

Tuck your butt and curl your lower back with your arms down. Then flip your palms with thumbs turned back as far as you can and reach down while you roll up one vertebra at a time until your body is in an upright position (counts one to four). Finish with one big shoulder roll

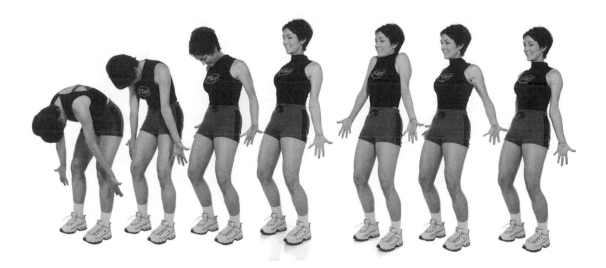

up and back (counts five to seven) with a final shoulder/neck stretch as your hands reach down (count eight).

Form Check Let your little finger drag along the side of your thighs to keep your hands in alignment with your shoulders.

Repeat entire Runner's Stretch with other leg—Steps 1 to 5, lunging with your left knee. It's important to take a water break after stretching.
    Proceed to Arm Sequence.

ARM SEQUENCE

T-Tapp Arm Sequence is a special series of comprehensive, compound muscle movements designed to create long, lean, dense muscles with teardrop-cut deltoid definition, giving you arms like a dancer's. Surprisingly, these movements look very simple, but once you try them you'll immediately feel the difference and realize that adding weights or increasing repetitions is never necessary to achieve results.

In addition to the sequence of movements, the secret to success with these arm exercises is that they maintain full fiber isometric activation while doing large muscle movement in linear alignment. The combination of these factors develops muscle density instead of muscle mass and uses much more fuel than traditional isotonic muscle movement.

However, don't make the common mistake of just going through the motions of movement. Since full fiber activation of your muscles takes more energy, fatigue can set in sooner than expected. It is better to do fewer repetitions with optimal form than to complete eight repetitions without maintaining isometric contractions or linear alignment.

Best of all, the stronger you get, the more challenging Arm Sequence will become and the less frequently you'll have to do it to maintain results. That's because application of T-Tapp techniques during movement empowers your body to maximize muscle mechanics. It takes muscle strength and neurokinetic flow to maintain isometric contractions along with flexibility to achieve range of motion while keeping your muscles tight. These two factors progressively build upon each other and enable continual challenge without the increase of repetitions or adding weight. If arms happen to be your target area of concern, Arm Sequence works well, done daily or in combination with Plié Sequence.

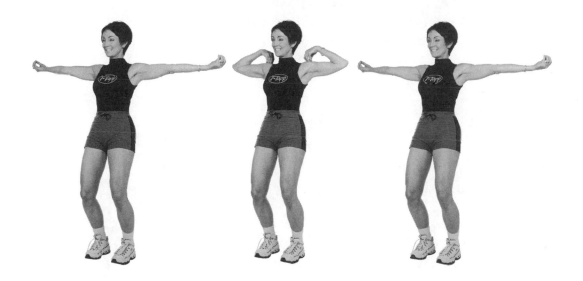

Step 1: Biceps Curls

It is important to establish correct lower body and upper body align-ment before starting Arm Sequence. For your lower body, assume the T-Tapp stance and maintain it at all times during arm movement. For your upper body, extend your arms straight out with your wrists, el-bows, and shoulders in alignment. Your hands should be in a doughnut position, behind your ears, and in alignment with your hips when seen from the side. Additionally, focus on keeping your hands in alignment with your hips. Now twist your thumbs back to keep your wrists level and to keep your elbows turned up to the ceiling. You should feel deep activation of every muscle in your back, especially your traps and lats. Now that your body is in alignment, let's get started!

While keeping your muscles tight, curl your hands in toward the tops of your shoulders without dropping your elbows (counts one and two). Then uncurl and extend your hands back out until your elbows and wrists are straight maintaining alignment between your elbows and shoulders (counts three and four).

Form Check Extend your hands all the way out until your knuckles are in alignment with your wrists.

Repeat for a total of eight repetitions, four counts each. Count each biceps curl as follows: curl in (counts one and two), extend out (counts three and four). Proceed to Step 2 without stopping.

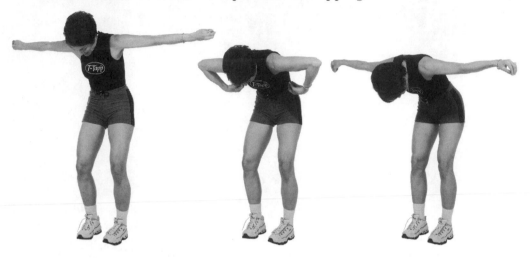

Step 2: Reverse Biceps Curls

Sequentially twist your arms—wrist, elbow, and shoulder—until your doughnut hands face the back wall. While twisting your arms, tuck your butt and slightly curl your spine until your head faces down.

Form Check Do not tuck your chin; it will create excess tension in your neck.

Then pull your elbows forward and up to maintain alignment with your shoulders as you curl your hands in toward your armpits with palms facing up. You should feel your triceps activate when you pull your elbows forward and up (counts one and two).

Then keep your elbows lifted up to maintain correct alignment with your shoulders as you uncurl and extend your hands all the way up until your knuckles are level with your elbows (counts three and four).

Form Check The palms of your doughnut hands should be facing the floor on count four, not the back wall like they do when you're twisting your arms into the setup position. Also do not relax your stomach.

Keep it tight by keeping your butt tucked and your knees pushing out at all times.

MOST COMMON MISTAKE

Letting your elbows aim back instead of pulling them forward will release activation of your triceps muscle and lessen results.

Repeat for a total of eight repetitions, four counts each. Count each reverse biceps curl as follows: curl in (counts one and two), extend out (counts three and four). Proceed to Step 3 without stopping.

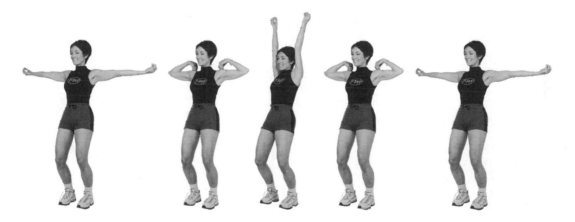

Step 3: Combo Curl-Ups

Uncurl your spine, pull your shoulders back, and flip your palms up to reestablish the starting position. Then, without releasing your elbow-to-shoulder alignment, curl your hands in and touch the tops of your shoulders (counts one and two). Then tuck your butt and bend your knees a little deeper as you reach above your head until your elbows are straight and in alignment with your shoulders and ears (counts three and four).

Form Check When reaching up, the palms of your doughnut hands should remain facing inward.

Then pull your elbows down, level with your shoulders, with your hands touching the tops of your shoulders (counts five and six).

Form Check When pulling your elbows down, keep them behind your ears and tighten your lats to help stabilize their position, so they do not drop lower than your shoulders.

Then, without releasing isometric contraction of your shoulders (traps and lats), extend your hands back out until they are level with your shoulders (counts seven and eight).

Repeat for a total of eight repetitions, eight counts each. Each combo curl-up is counted as follows: curl in (counts one and two), reach up (counts three and four), curl in (counts five and six), extend out (counts seven and eight). Proceed to Step 4 without stopping.

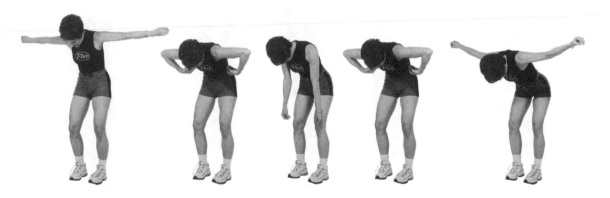

Step 4: Reverse Combo Curl-Ups

Repeat counts one and two of Step 2. Then pull your shoulders back and tighten your lats at the same time you extend your hands down until your elbows are straight. Your elbows and wrists should be in alignment with your shoulders (counts three and four).

MOST COMMON MISTAKE

Relaxing your shoulders as you reach down inactivates upper back and abdominal muscles. Always tighten your lats to keep your shoulders back.

Then pull your elbows forward as you curl your hands back up toward your armpits (counts five and six).

Form Check When curling hands up, aim to the middle of your armpit or side seam of your shirt to help keep your hands in correct alignment at armpit. The most common mistake is aiming your hands to the front of your armpit (pectoral muscles) instead of the middle of your armpit (triceps and lats).

Then, without releasing isometric contraction of your shoulders (traps and lats), extend your hands back out until they are level with your shoulders (counts seven and eight).

Repeat for a total of eight repetitions, eight counts each. Count each reverse combo curl as follows: reverse curl in (counts one and two), reach down (counts three and four), curl in (counts five and six), and uncurl out (counts seven and eight). Proceed to Step 5 without stopping.

Step 5: Clap-Pull-Clap-Release

While maintaining your lower body in the T-Tapp stance and while keeping your shoulders in alignment with your hips, do the following clap sequence to release muscle tension and toxins. Straighten your elbows and clap your hands in front of your body (count one), then pull your elbows back with elbows up (count two), then clap again to the front (count three), and with momentum, try to clap your hands behind with your arms straight (count four). It's okay if your hands don't touch in the back—just keep your arms as straight as possible to achieve results.

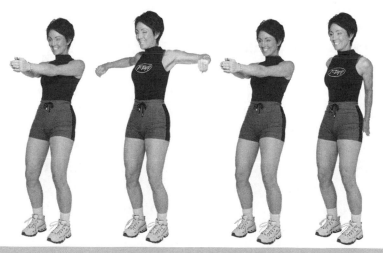

Repeat for a total of four repetitions, four counts each. Count each clap-pull-clap-release sequence as follows: clap in front (count one), pull elbows (count two), clap in front (count three), and clap behind (count four). This sequence should feel good, so if you have extra muscle fatigue and/or tension, feel free to do an extra set. Proceed to Step 6 without stopping.

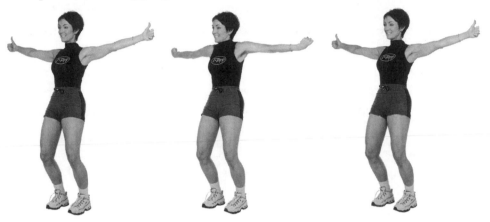

Step 6: Hitchhikers

Extend your arms out at shoulder level with your hands in fists and thumbs up. Your hands should be in alignment with your hips, shoulders, and ears when viewed from the side. Continue to maintain the T-Tapp stance with your shoulders back and in alignment with your hips at all times.

Keep your elbows straight while you twist with your wrists, thumbs pointing forward, down and back as far as you can while maintaining linear alignment of your arms (counts one and two). Then twist with your wrists to return your thumbs to the front, up and as far back as you can (counts three and four).

Form Check Keep your elbows straight and in alignment with your shoulders and wrists while twisting.

Repeat for a total of four repetitions, four counts each. Count each hitchhiker as follows: twist down (counts one and two), twist back (counts three and four). Proceed to Step 7 without stopping.

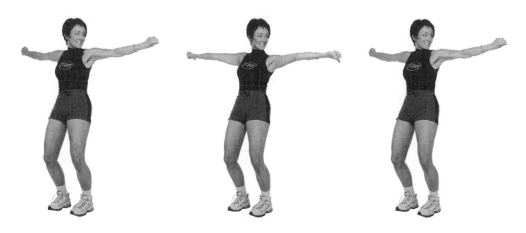

Step 7: Hitchhikers Left and Right

Now look to your left as far as you can, maintaining linear alignment of your shoulder to hip as well as your shoulder, elbow, and wrist, and repeat hitchhikers four more times.

Form Check Keep your head straight while looking to your left. Do not allow the top of your head to tilt back, a common error.

Then look to your right as far as you can and repeat hitchhikers four more times.

Repeat for a total of four repetitions to the left and four repetitions to the right, four counts each. Count each hitchhiker left and right as follows: twist down (counts one and two), twist back (counts three and four). Proceed to Step 8 without stopping.

Step 8: Hitchhikers Part 2 Setup

Let your muscles between your shoulder blades relax as you tilt your body over and drop your hands down in 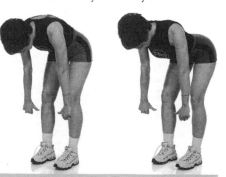 alignment with your shoulders as shown in my image on the left. Your fingers should be curled in and your thumbs should be pointing at each other.

Inhale big (counts one to four), and during the exhale, pull your shoulders back and arch your butt up to stabilize your shoulders, spine, and hips (counts five to eight).

Form Check Your shoulders do not have to be level with your hips, but do not have them lower than your hips.

Proceed to Step 9 without stopping.

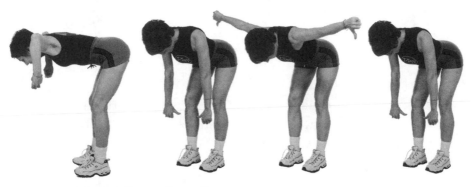

Step 9: Hitchhikers Part 2

Then pull your elbows forward and up as high as you can (counts one and two).

Form Check Maintain linear alignment between your wrists and elbows for optimal results.

Then punch your arms down without releasing shoulder muscles (counts three and four).

Form Check Tighten your lats to pull your shoulders back at the same time you punch your arms down to help stabilize your shoulders.

Then extend your arms straight out to shoulder height with thumbs pointing toward the floor (counts five and six).

Form Check Do not use momentum to swing arms up. Use your muscles and tighten your lats to control arm movement to stop at shoulder height.

Then bring your arms back down without bending your elbows and without releasing your shoulders (counts seven and eight).

Repeat for a total of eight repetitions, eight counts each.

Count each hitchhiker part 2 as follows: bring elbows up (counts one and two), punch down (counts three and four), arms up (counts five and six), and arms down (counts seven and eight). Proceed to Step 10 without stopping.

Step 10: Head Rocks

Place your hands on the outside of your calves (not ankles) and relax your upper body. Feel the gravitational pull on your head and relax (counts one and two), then inhale and exhale to help release any muscle tension (counts three and four). Then, while tightening your butt, push your hands into your calves and pull your shoulders back for isometric spinal support (counts five and six). Then do another inhale and exhale while maintaining isometric contractions for deeper stretch (counts seven and eight). Now gently rock your head four times without any other body movement. Proceed to Step 11 without stopping.

Step 11: Spine Roll-Up and Shoulder Roll

Tuck your butt and curl your lower back with your arms down. Then flip your palms with your thumbs turned back as far as you can and

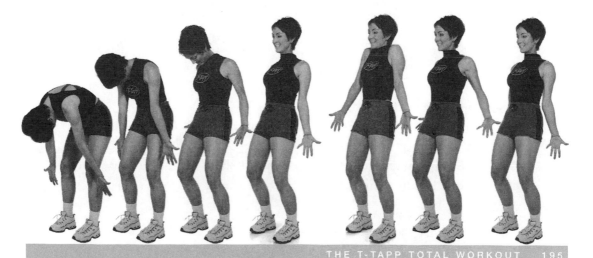

reach down while you roll up one vertebra at a time until your body is in an upright position (counts one to four). Finish with one big shoulder roll, up and back (counts five to seven) with one final shoulder and neck stretch as you reach your hands down (count eight). Proceed to Step 12 without stopping.

Step 12: Clap-Pull-Clap-Release
Repeat Step 5 (see details and photo reference page 191). Then proceed to Step 13 without stopping.

Step 13: Arm Stretch Part 1
Push your right elbow toward your left shoulder while reaching back with your right hand toward your spine. Try to maintain linear alignment between your right elbow and right shoulder. Then inhale (counts one and two) and during the exhale increase pressure on your right elbow for optimal stretch (counts three and four). While maintaining constant pressure on your right elbow, pat yourself on your back four times with your right hand (counts five to eight).

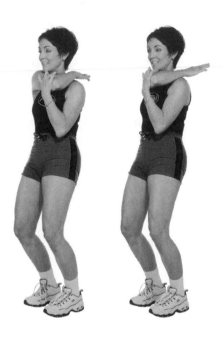

Form Check Keep your shoulders back, butt tucked, and knees pushing out at all times.

Repeat on the other side. Then proceed to Step 14 without stopping.

Step 14: Arm Stretch Part 2
Keep your lower body in T-Tapp stance and put your hands up behind your head. Use your left hand to pull your right hand down and your right elbow up in alignment with your right shoulder, and inhale and exhale while holding this position for four counts.

Form Check During inhale (counts one and two), expand your rib cage to the best of your ability, and during the exhale (counts three and four), increase the pull on your right hand and pull your ribs in to the best of your ability.

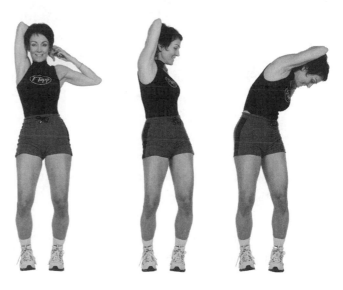

Inhale again (counts five and six), and during the exhale, push your right knee out at the same time you twist your upper body to your left (counts seven and eight). Then increase the intensity of your right knee pushing out and the intensity of your butt tuck as you tilt your upper body over to the left and toward the floor (counts one to four). Then inhale big and exhale bigger while holding this position (counts five to eight).

Form Check Keep your weight equally distributed, but really push your right knee out and pull your ribs in during the exhale. You should feel the stretch in your lower back increase when you tuck and push out more with your right knee.

Proceed to Step 15 without stopping.

Step 15: Arm Stretch Part 3

Extend your upper body back up facing to the left (counts one and two). Then turn your upper body to face forward (counts three and

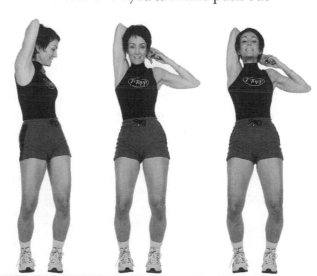

four). Then push your head back into your right arm for optimal stretch (counts five to eight). This should feel good.

Release and repeat arm stretch parts 1, 2, and 3 to the other side. Follow form and details in Steps 13, 14, and 15.

Now take a water break and proceed to Step 16.

Step 16: Butterflies Part 1

Extend your arms out at shoulder level with palms up and your thumbs pointing back as far as you can.

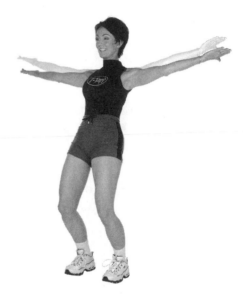

Form Check Reach away with your hands like someone is pulling your arms. When doing this, you should feel greater isometric contraction, not only in your arms, but also in your back. Your lower body should be in the T-Tapp stance at all times.

Now, without bending your elbows, move your arms up and down approximately six inches for a total of eight repetitions. Proceed to Step 17 without stopping.

Step 17: Butterflies Part 2

Bend your knees a little deeper, tuck your butt a bit harder, and keep your shoulders back as you butterfly your arms a bit bigger. Lift your extended arms (keep reaching away) up and down from your shoulder to your waist for a total of eight repetitions (two counts each).

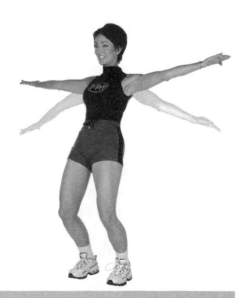

Form Check Tighten your lats to stabilize your arm movement to stop at shoulder height. Control your arm movement without momentum.

Proceed to Step 18 without stopping.

Step 18: Butterflies Part 3

Bend your knees even deeper, tuck a little more, and lean back a little bit as you continue to butterfly your arms all the way down until your hands are beside your body (counts one and two) and all the way back up until they are level with your shoulders (counts three and four).

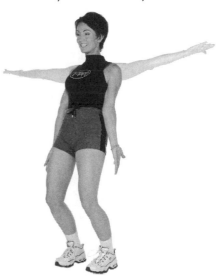

Form Check Press your chest forward and pull your shoulders back as you reach down to the sides of your body. Focus to turn your thumbs back as far as you can each time you reach down.

Repeat for a total of eight repetitions (four counts each). Shake out your arms and proceed to Step 19.

Step 19: Lateral Lat Pulls

Assume the T-Tapp stance to maintain isometric isolation of your lower body while moving your arms. Then extend your arms at shoulder level with your hands in a doughnut position with palms up. Make sure your wrists are in alignment with your shoulders and behind your ears. Now that you're in correct position, let's get started.

Inhale first (counts one and two) while your arms are extended. Then, while exhaling, pull your elbows down to the sides of your body with your elbows pushing forward and your hands pulling back (counts three to six).

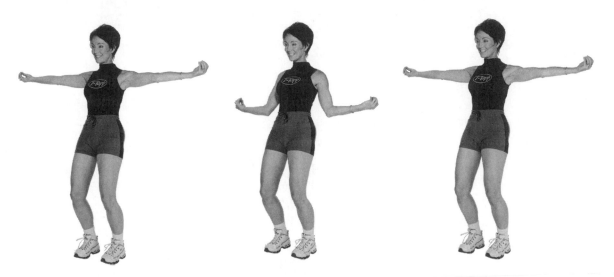

Form Check Maintain alignment of your elbows and hands to your shoulders or ears (as viewed from the side) during the pull, and exhale all the way until you feel your ribs pull in. You should feel deep isometric tightening within all your back muscles, especially the lats.

Then inhale as you bring your arms back out in alignment with your shoulders (counts seven and eight).

Repeat for a total of eight repetitions, eight counts each. Count each lateral lat pull as follows: inhale and reach out (counts one and two), exhale and pull down (counts three to six), and then inhale and reach out (counts seven and eight). Proceed to Step 20 without stopping.

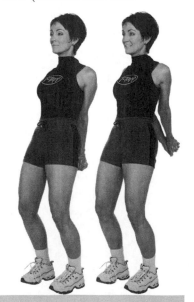

Step 20: Arm Pumps

Clasp your hands behind your back (or use a towel, as described in Primary Back Stretch). Twist your elbows in to help pull your shoulders back and lift/touch your arms to the base of your spine for a total of four arm pumps without moving your shoulders. Proceed to Step 21 without stopping.

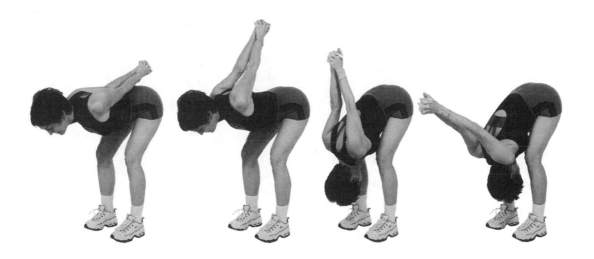

Step 21: Horizontal Arm Pumps and Ostrich Roll

With your hands behind your back and your lower body in the T-Tapp stance, bend at your waist and assume a flat back position. Then arch your butt up and pull your shoulders back to stabilize your body position. Do four more lift/touch arm pumps to the best of your ability without moving your spine.

Then continue to bend over for a full spinal stretch while maintaining the same arm position (with or without a towel) to your own personal max. Hold this position and tuck your chin as you inhale (counts one and two). You should feel increased stretching throughout your torso and back. Then relax your head as you exhale (counts three and four). Repeat inhale (counts five and six) and exhale (counts seven and eight) and release your arms. Proceed to Step 22 without stopping.

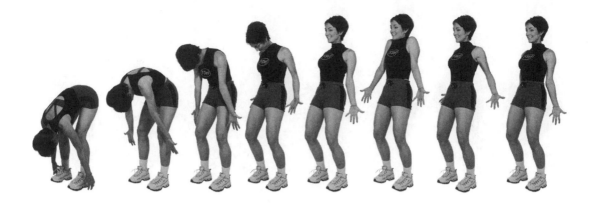

Step 22: Final Spine Roll-Up with Shoulder Roll

Tuck your butt, flip your palms, and reach down as you continue to roll up one vertebra at a time until your body is in an upright position (counts one to four). Finish with one big shoulder roll up, back, and down with your thumbs pointing back as far as you can and in alignment behind your ears.

Take a water break and proceed to Torso Twist.

TORSO TWIST

After finishing Arm Sequence, your back and shoulder muscles will welcome the stretch and release of muscle tension they will receive during Torso Twist. This exercise is designed to trim your torso, increase core strength and flexibility, and provide lymphatic release in the thoracic area of your spine. Although it appears simple, Torso Twist involves comprehensive, isometric muscle movement along with comprehensive, compound large muscle movement to help isolate your upper body from your lower body for ultimate body sculpting and inch loss. The action of tucking your butt while twisting in combination with keeping your supportive knee bent in KLT will challenge your core and activate abdominal muscles to the max. So tuck, tighten, and twist those inches away with Torso Twist!

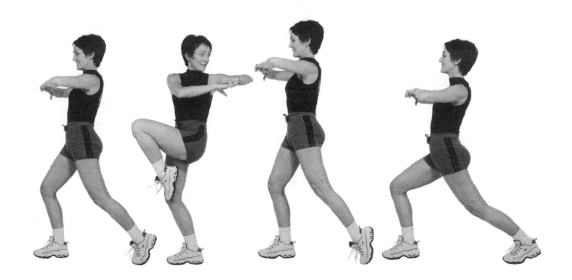

Step 1: Complete Movement

Step back into a moderate lunge position with your feet hip width apart (not a straight line) and your right knee bent in KLT position. Your upper body should be straight with your shoulders square to the sides and pulled back in alignment with your hips. Now press your hands together just below your collarbone for full activation of your back muscles, especially your lats. At the same time you press, tuck your butt until you feel your lower back muscles tighten and push your chest forward. Every muscle in your back should be equally tight with full activation along your spine. The weight of your body should be completely in your right leg and your left foot should be straight (no turnout).

Form Check Keep your back muscles tight with your butt tucked and shoulders in alignment with your hips at all times to support your spine and receive optimal results. Proceed to Step 2.

Step 2: Tuck Twist

Tuck your butt as you lift your left knee and twist it to your right side. You should feel your stomach muscles tighten when you tuck and lift at the same time. While your lower body is twisting to the right, your upper body twists to the left with your left elbow in perfect alignment with your left shoulder. Your eyes should focus on your left elbow during the twist so you can achieve a complete spinal twist in your upper body. Your range of motion will improve as your muscles develop more strength and flexibility, so always twist to your personal max. You should aim to achieve a twist with your left knee facing in complete opposition to your left elbow.

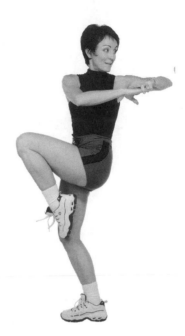

Form Check Pull your ribs in and drop your right elbow while you twist, so you can maintain alignment of your shoulder, spine, and hips. Never let your left elbow drop lower than your left shoulder. It is better to aim a bit high than to be too low. Linear alignment between your left elbow and left shoulder is important not only for optimal results but also (and primarily) for spinal safety.

Proceed to Step 3.

MOST COMMON MISTAKES

In addition to dropping your elbow lower than your shoulder, another common mistake is straightening your supportive knee during the twist. Always keep your knee bent and pushing out into KLT to stabilize your lower body and support your spine.

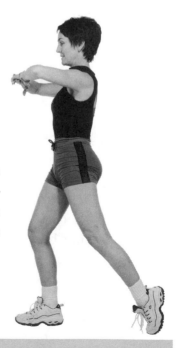

Step 3

While maintaining shoulder/hip alignment with your butt tucked, twist back to your starting position. Your elbows should return to a level position with hands pressing against each other. Proceed to Step 4.

Step 4: KLT Drop Heel

Then drop your left heel and push your right knee out more as you lower your body. This simultaneous action might cause you to lose your balance because it creates core challenge. But bobbling is good.

Form Check The movement of your body should be up and down with your spine centered. Do not shift your weight into your left leg, and keep your left foot straight. Turnout of your left knee will inactivate the muscles that attach to your left hip and lessen results.

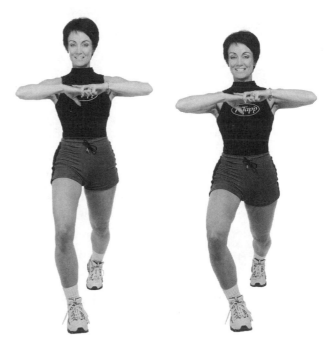

Repeat for a total of eight repetitions, four counts each. Count each torso twist as follows: tuck twist left knee over (count one), twist back touching toe (count two), drop left heel and hold (counts three and four).

Repeat on the other side, Steps 1–4 with your right knee twisting, for a total of eight repetitions. Then repeat once more on each side for a total of two sets.

Proceed to Step Lift Sequence without stopping, or take a water break if needed.

STEP LIFT SEQUENCE

Step Lift Sequence is designed to raise your heart rate and to help your body eliminate excess lactic acid. The aerobic and lymphatic nature of this cardiokinetic sequence also boosts your body's ability to burn fat. The combination of body sculpting, inch loss, cardiac conditioning, and core movement gives this seemingly simple exercise the ability to deliver big results from head to toe. I consider Step Lift Sequence to be a little mini-max workout all by itself. Max results in minimal time—it's perfect for those who have no time to lose, just inches and fat. So step away and discover how less is more with T-Tapp.

Step 1: Step Lift Part 1

Extend the heel of your right hand level at shoulder height with your knuckles pulled back and your wrist in alignment behind your ear. Your left hand should be below your waist with your thumb pushing into your back and your fingers off your body. Now pull your left elbow back. You should feel every muscle tighten in your back and alignment of your left shoulder improve. The weight of your body should be on your left leg with your left knee bent in KLT. Your right foot should be touching the floor with your right knee also bent in KLT. Then inhale big (counts one and two), and during the exhale, push your thumb into your back and pull your shoulders down to fully stretch your traps (counts three and four). Now you're ready to begin.

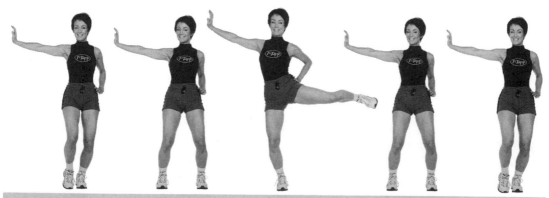

Step out and shift your weight into your right leg (count one). Then tuck your butt and push your right knee out as you lift your left leg with toes facing forward and/or slightly turned in (count two).

MOST COMMON MISTAKE

Allowing your left foot to point up as you lift your leg works your thigh muscles rather than your core. *Tip:* Push your left heel down, pull up your toes, and slightly turn your left knee as you turn in your foot to stabilize your foot position and optimize results. This little tip helps your body battle cellulite, too!

Drop your left leg until your weight is equally distributed with both of your knees bent in KLT (count three). Then bring your right foot back in and touch the floor (count four) with your weight shifting into your right leg. Both of your knees should be bent and in KLT position.

Repeat for a total of eight repetitions, four counts each. Count step lift part 1 as follows: step out (count one), lift left leg (count two), leg down (count three), and step together (count four).

Proceed to Step 2 without stopping.

Step 2: Step Lift Part 2

Flip your right palm up and repeat Step 1, pointing your thumb back as far as you can.

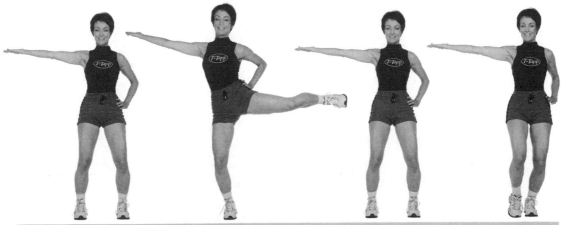

Repeat for a total of eight repetitions, four counts each. Count each step lift part 2 as follows: step out (count one), lift left leg (count two), leg down (count three), and step together (count four).

Proceed to Step 3 without stopping.

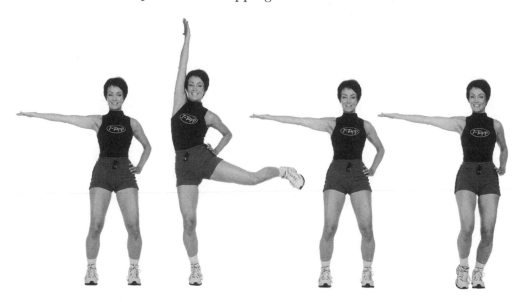

Step 3: Step Lift Part 3

Maintain right palm up and repeat Step 2 sequence except for count two. Do count two as follows: at the same time you push your right knee out and lift your left leg, bring your right arm up until your right hand is in alignment with your right shoulder.

Form Check Your right arm and hand should reach up rather than just laterally move into correct position. Furthermore, at the same time you reach, increase the intensity of your butt tuck and push your left thumb into your back. Feel the greater rib-to-hip stretch? This will optimize your results.

MOST COMMON MISTAKE

Allowing your right elbow to bend and/or bringing your right arm across your body instead of keeping it aligned with the right shoulder inactivates muscle attachments and creates isotonic movement with momentum. *Tip:* Tuck and tighten all your muscles at the same time you reach up to help you prevent momentum follow through. This also will help you establish better kinetic awareness of where your body is in space. Mind/body awareness improves quickly with T-Tapp.

Repeat for a total of eight repetitions, four counts each. Count each step lift part 3 as follows: step out (count one), lift right arm and left leg (count two), lower right arm and left leg (count three), and step together (count four).

Repeat entire sequence on the other side, lifting with your right leg, without stopping.

Then proceed to Step 4.

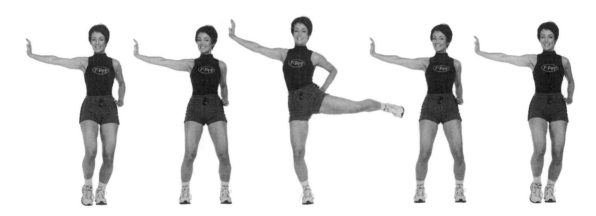

Step 4: Step Lift Part 4

Repeat Step 1 for a total of eight repetitions, four counts each.

Proceed to Step 5 without stopping.

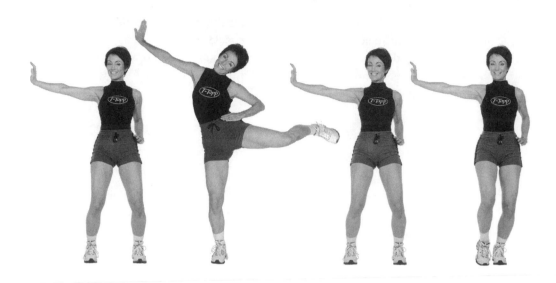

Step 5: Step Lift Part 5

Repeat Step 1 sequence except for count two. Do count two as follows: at the same time you push your right knee out and lift your left leg, tilt your upper body toward your left.

Form Check Keep the muscles in your right arm tight, with your hand pulling back as much as you can. It's okay if your right hand lifts higher than your shoulder, but it's important to keep it in linear alignment behind your ear. Keep your shoulders back and in alignment with your hips so your upper body tilts in lateral alignment. *Tip:* Increase the intensity of your butt tuck and right knee pushing out to help you lift your left leg in alignment. By now your muscles are fatigued and your body will look for the path of least resistance. That's usually when your body prefers to lift your leg slightly to the front instead of staying in lateral alignment to your shoulders. Focus on keeping your left ankle in alignment with your left hip and shoulder (as seen from the side).

Repeat for a total of eight repetitions, four counts each. Count each step lift part 5 as follows: step out (count one), tilt upper body and lift left leg (count two), straighten tilt and lower left leg (count three), and step together (count four).

Repeat Step 5 on the other side without stopping, for a total of eight repetitions, four counts each.

Proceed to Step 6 without stopping.

Step 6: Head Rocks

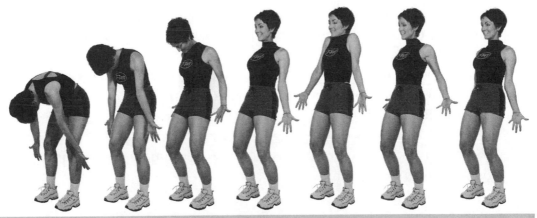

Place your hands on the outside of your calves (not ankles) and relax your upper body while you inhale (counts one and two) and exhale (counts three and four). Then push your hands into your calves and push your knees out and tighten your butt to optimize lymphatic function as well as stretch your hamstrings, but do not tighten your shoulders this time. Gently rock your head four times (counts one to four). Then tighten your shoulders for isometric spinal support and repeat another four head rocks (counts five to eight). Repeat another inhale (counts one and two) and exhale (counts three and four). Proceed to Step 7 without stopping.

Step 7: Final Spinal Roll-Up with Shoulder Roll

Tuck your butt, flip your palms, and reach down as you continue to roll up one vertebra at a time until your body is in an upright position (counts one to four). Finish with one big shoulder roll with your thumbs pointing back as far as you can and in alignment behind your ears.

Take a water break and proceed to Lawn Mowers.

LAWN MOWERS

I created Lawn Mowers to help your body optimize core development with strength, flexibility, spinal stretch from rib to hip, and lymphatic function. Its unique combination of lateral movement along with twisting your spine in opposition with isometric isolation develops muscle density with girdle strength. Not only does this help your body to tighten, tone, and cinch in your midsection, but it also assists your body's ability to burn fat and eliminate any stored toxins. Many consider Lawn Mowers to be a signature move for a trimmer torso, especially Short Torso body types.

Lawn Mowers target the thoracic area of your spine, an area that is often overlooked and underused during daily activity. This movement sequence works well and feels good in releasing any muscle tension along your spine from extended isometric contractions required for maintaining linear alignment during large muscle movement.

Best of all, it's the last move from the Total Workout.

Step 1: Lawn Mower Stretch

Assume the T-Tapp stance. Then twist your upper body to the left until your shoulders are square to the side. Now tuck and push your right knee out more as you reach down with your upper body, hands aiming to the back of your knee and fingertips pointing to the heel of your shoe. You should feel an extended spinal stretch down your right side.

Then, shift your body weight to be a little more in your left leg and relax your head. Hold this position (counts one to four), then inhale and exhale (counts five to eight).

Inhale again as you pull your right elbow up to the ceiling (counts one to four) and exhale as you maintain your body in a lateral tilt (counts five to eight).

Form Check Relax your head when you exhale and let the weight of your body stretch your muscles.

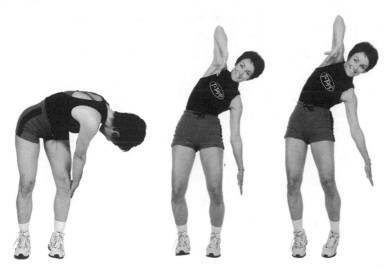

Then increase the intensity of your butt tuck, as well as how far you push your left knee out, as you reach up higher with your right elbow and reach down with your left hand (counts one and two). Then release your reach, but maintain your body position (counts three and four) and hold (counts five to eight).

Form Check Your right elbow should be in alignment with your right shoulder with your right palm facing out and your left arm should be hanging down with your left palm facing in toward the center of your body. It's okay if you lift your left heel off the floor when you reach up higher with your elbow, but it's very important to keep your right leg stable with both knees bent and pushing out to KLT.

MOST COMMON MISTAKES

Pulling your right elbow back instead of up will pull your right shoulder out of alignment, as shown in the photo. This inactivates muscles in your upper back and can cause strain to your shoulder and spine. Another mistake, as shown in the second photo, is not bringing your left shoulder forward to be in alignment with your left hip when you pull your right elbow up. This inactivates muscles in your lower back and lessens results. Focus on keeping your shoulders square to the front and back in alignment with

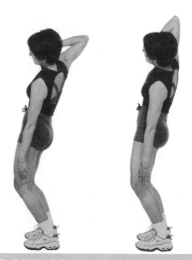

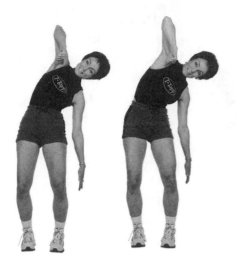

your hips whenever your upper body is in a lateral tilt position, not only for optimal results but also to protect and provide spinal support.

Repeat for a total of three repetitions, eight counts each. Count each stretch as follows: tuck and reach elbow up higher (counts one and two), release (counts three and four) and hold (counts five to eight). Proceed to Step 2 without stopping.

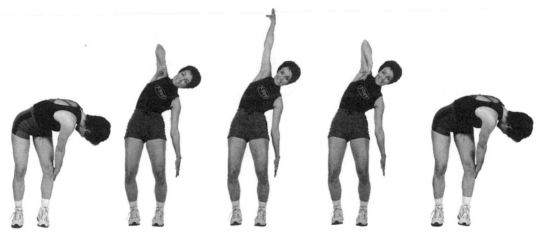

Step 2: Lawn Mowers

Tuck your butt and push your right knee out as you bring your right arm back down and over to your left side to reestablish the starting position (counts one to four). Inhale and exhale while holding this position (counts five to eight).

Then, while maintaining your lower body in T-Tapp stance, pull your right elbow up (counts one and two) and extend your right hand until your arm is straight with palm facing out (counts three and four). Then bend your elbow, but keep it up and in alignment with your right shoulder while you bring your right hand down (counts five and six). Then return to the start position (counts seven and eight).

Repeat for a total of eight repetitions, eight counts each.

Count as follows: right elbow up (counts one and two), extend arm straight (counts three and four), bring hand down with elbow up (counts five and six), and return to start position (counts seven and eight). On the eighth repetition, for counts five through eight reach up and out with your arm until it is down by your right side. Then proceed to Step 3 without stopping.

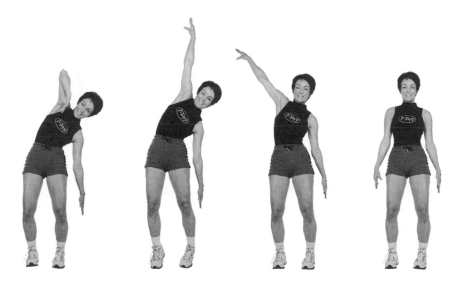

Form Check Increase the intensity of your tuck and extend the distance between your right rib to hip to your personal max during reach (counts five to eight) to receive best results. Do not straighten your knees.

Step 3: Head Rocks

Place your hands on the outside of your calves and relax your upper body while you inhale (counts one and two) and exhale (counts three and four). Then push your hands into your calves and push your knees out to tighten the muscles in your upper back and gently rock your head four times (counts one to four). Now tighten your butt to increase isometric activation of your lower back and thighs and do four more head rocks (counts five to eight). Inhale again (counts one and two) and exhale (counts three and four).

Proceed to Step 4 without stopping.

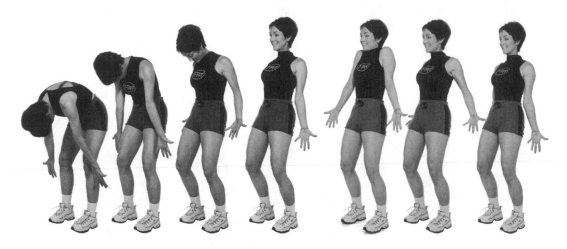

Step 4: Spinal Roll-Up and Shoulder Roll

Then tuck your butt, flip your palms, and reach down as you continue to roll up one vertebra at a time until your body is in an upright position (counts one to four). Finish with one big shoulder roll with your thumbs pointing back as far as you can while maintaining alignment behind your ears.

Form Check Keep your hands below your hips while doing the shoulder roll.

Repeat Steps 1 to 4 on the other side without stopping.

YOU DID IT

You did it! That completes the Total Workout. Take a water break and have a great day!

6

The God-Made, Man-Made Food Plan

Remember when you were a kid and could get away with eating almost anything—even junk food? Back then, you moved your body a lot more, plus you had better digestion, assimilation, and elimination. Good news: T-Tapp not only gets you moving again, it *rebuilds* those basic body functions and turns back time, so you can eat, cheat, and get away with it!

Do I restrict calories? Definitely not. I have a hearty appetite and typically consume 2,000 to 3,000 calories daily with plenty of treats. Do I T-Tapp every day? No! When I'm getting ready for a fitness event, I'll do a four-day boot camp, but then I might go a week or so (sometimes longer) without doing anything but Primary Back Stretch and Hoe Downs. I've even gone up to six weeks without exercising or changing my diet, but usually my back pain returns (along with extra inches) to put me back on track.

As I said earlier in this book, I don't believe in dieting. In fact, during your first few weeks of T-Tapping, I don't recommend changing your eating habits at all. I've found it's far better for you (and your body) to concentrate on one new change at a time. So, instead of worrying about altering your food intake, focus on moving your body in the special T-Tapp sequence.

Once you feel comfortable T-Tapping, I do encourage you to satisfy your hunger with healthy foods, but I still don't advocate dieting per se. To me, the very word *diet* means deprivation, and study after study shows that cutting out foods you love—and crave—only makes you more likely to overeat.

Given my philosophy on dieting, why include a food plan in this book? For starters, I recognize that many people are focused on what the scale says, and this plan will help you drop pounds in addition to the inches you'll lose with the T-Tapp workout. I also realize that telling you to give up your favorite foods may very well set you up for failure. When researchers at the University of Rochester Medical School recently studied 450 women, they found that most abandoned their diets after a single slip-up. That's why controlled cheating is so effective, and why this food plan enables you to splurge every third day—so you're more likely to stay on track and lose more inches as well as weight.

I definitely don't advocate diets that are stingy with calories. These can make you feel lousy and way too sluggish to T-Tapp. Super-low-carb diets also concern me. In fact, I believe these can be dangerous because they don't allow proper conversion of glucose to energy. When deprived of carbs, your body will use protein for energy, thus robbing protein of its primary job: building and repairing tissue.

In addition, studies have shown that if you totally eliminate carbs from your diet, the body's metabolic rate changes. Granted, this may allow you to lose weight initially, but once carbs are reintroduced, that weight quickly returns, and most people gain even *more* weight.

"Many of today's popular diets are not optimally balanced for long-term health and well-being," agrees Margaret Merrifield, M.D.,

C.C.F.E., medical director at the Center for Health and Wellbeing in Richland, Washington. "Besides, research shows that the building—or recovery—of lean muscle tissue is the most efficient way to change body size and shape." In other words, when you use exercises such as T-Tapp to rev up your metabolism and build muscle density, you don't need to restrict calories to lose fat.

Studies have also proven that exercise is more important than diet when it comes to weight management. Of course, we all know that a healthy diet combined with exercising is the best way to look trim and feel terrific. And with T-Tapp, you can do it all.

That's why I have created what I call the God-Made, Man-Made Food Plan—to help you lose weight in addition to inches. The good news is that you don't have to give up any of the foods you love—even "bad" (or what I call "man-made") carbs. Instead, this plan literally trains your body to process man-made carbs, and that will keep your weight under control.

Again, this is no fad diet. You will never count calories or points, and I won't ask you to measure food portions. You eat whenever you're hungry, and no food is off-limits. Think of this food plan as a common-sense approach to eating that will make you healthier and at the same time enable you to control your weight *without* feeling deprived. With the God-Made, Man-Made Food Plan, you're simply helping your body help itself digest and assimilate the nutrients it needs, which are the building blocks for your body to build muscles as well as to burn fat and calories.

I developed the God-Made, Man-Made Food Plan while working in Europe. I was always curious about why so many Americans struggled with their weight, while in those days most Europeans did not. I knew Europeans were far less dependent on their cars and walked more, but they also seemed to break every diet rule. Granted, things have changed in recent years with the introduction of so many American fast-food restaurants abroad. And just like their American counterparts, many of today's European children lead sedentary lifestyles, preferring to play video games instead of exercising.

Nevertheless, Europeans continue to eat plenty of fats and carbs and don't seem to pack on the extra pounds as Americans do. Think about it. The French gobble up croissants, Italians eat pasta with rich sauces, and Germans are crazy for cheese. Europeans also tend to eat late at night and drink wine. So how do so many of them manage to stay svelte?

For starters, it's not uncommon for Europeans to go to the market every day. As a result, they tend to eat fresher foods with no preservatives—foods the body recognizes and can easily handle. Americans, on the other hand, have a tendency to shop for foods with a longer shelf life. And as I always say, the more preservatives in your food, the more you preserve on your butt and gut.

Elizabeth Koepke

"Eating healthy has brought me so many benefits!"

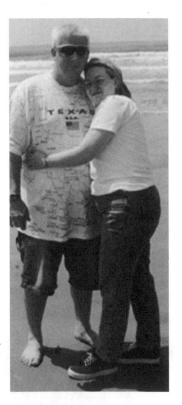

Two years ago, I had a wake-up call. I looked in the mirror one morning and was shocked at the stretch marks I had across my lower abdomen—not from pregnancy, but from constant weight gain over five years. I knew I had to make changes in my life or I would continue to get bigger. In the past, I had tried to lose weight through different exercise programs and going to the gym, but after a few months—with no visible results—I'd give up.

I realized I had to make a lifestyle change and began looking into different ways of exercising and eating. Through T-Tapp I learned of the God-Made, Man-Made Food Plan. Everything made sense to me. In August 2002, I began to follow this plan and exercise at the gym. I saw some results. In the fall, I started T-Tapping instead of going to the gym and saw even greater results. By January, I had shrunk from a size fourteen to a size eight.

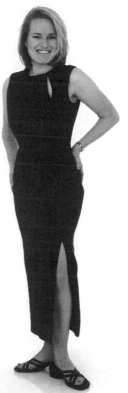

Following the God-Made, Man-Made Food Plan has also improved my health. My periods have gone from long and irregular to short and consistently regular. Two years ago, I was taking antacids daily, but since making this lifestyle change, I haven't had heartburn once!

I need to keep my body healthy to prevent heart disease. My family has a history of high cholesterol and high blood pressure. It is important to me to take preventative measures against these health problems, and by eating the T-Tapp way and doing the T-Tapp workout, it's easy to do that!

Processed foods typically bear little resemblance to foods in their whole, natural forms. They are manufactured, "value-added" products that are often stripped of vital nutrients and laden with excessive amounts of salt, sugar, and fat as well as synthetic flavors and chemicals. What's more, when you heat up processed foods, the heat often destroys any nutrients that may have been left.

Many so-called diet foods aren't much better. "Lite" foods are almost always made with sucrose, bleached white flour, or flavor enhancers that are known to trigger hormones that can stimulate overeating. In contrast, fresh, unpackaged, and unprocessed foods provide more fiber and healthy fat, both of which trigger anti-hunger hormones.

If you think about it, our bodies are natural (or God-made). So it makes perfect sense that our bodies instinctively know what to do with fresh, natural God-made foods versus foods that are processed or altered in a laboratory (man-made) for longer shelf life. If nothing else, it's going to be harder for your body to recognize, digest, and eliminate man-made foods—and that alone can affect weight loss and even contribute to weight gain.

Research proves this to be true. Recent studies from Tufts University found that subjects who ate so-called diet foods were much more likely to overeat than those who ate fresh foods such as those favored by Europeans. And when scientists at Brigham and Women's Hospital and

Harvard Medical School put test subjects on a European-style diet versus a low-fat plan, they uncovered some surprising results: Euro-style dieters lost weight, while low-fat dieters gained!

These findings don't surprise me a bit. Most diet foods are loaded with preservatives and additives, which don't satisfy your hunger the way whole foods do. In fact, they often create a nutritional imbalance that makes you eat more, because you end up craving whatever you're missing.

Traditionally, Europeans have also eaten slowly. Folks in Italy and France are notorious for their lengthy meals. They take time to savor every bite, to converse with family and friends, and to digest whatever they are eating. In contrast, Americans tend to crave immediate gratification. We pick up fast food at drive-through windows and eat on the go. Or we talk and gobble food at the same time. Big mistake. Anytime you wolf down food, your hormones don't have enough time to send signals to your brain that enough is enough. As a result, you overeat—and often feel bloated and miserable afterward.

Europeans drink a lot of wine as well, and the health benefits of this beverage—particularly red wine—are legendary. Surely you've heard all about the research that says drinking red wine in moderation can keep your heart healthy. Now, new studies are finding that sipping one to two glasses of red wine a day may also decrease your sensitivity to insulin, so your body doesn't pump out high levels of this fat-storage hormone. So if you are going to drink, make it red, which is my beverage of choice, regardless of whether I'm eating meat or fish.

While creating the God-Made, Man-Made Food Plan, I studied many existing dietary plans. I've always believed in getting a balance of nutrients and limiting processed foods as much as possible. Our bodies need protein to build muscle and regulate hormones that control appetite. We need fat to fuel the brain, and yes, we need carbs to give us energy (a necessary prerequisite for T-Tapping). In fact, this food plan is loosely based on Johns Hopkins Medical Center research, which states that women need 55 percent of their calories from carbs to prevent bone density loss.

Jenny Russell

"I'm eating more than I ever have—and staying fit and fabulous!"

I have struggled with my weight all my life. People would always say to me, "You're not fat; you're just a little chunky." Since my teenage years, I've had a history of dieting and have tried everything to lose weight: the cabbage soup diet, the grapefruit diet, the Atkins diet, the weight loss magnets, and everything in between.

I began doing the T-Tapp workout in September 2001 at size twelve. By December, I had dropped to a size nine or ten. I kept doing the workout two to three times each week, but sometimes I managed just once a week. By September 2002, I had dropped to a size six.

I began T-Tapp's God-Made, Man-Made Food Plan in September 2002, and it changed my life. Since I have a nutrition degree and have taken lots of science courses in college, the information made a lot of sense to me. I had so much energy, and I loved eating what I wanted on my man-made days. I even went through a period of high stress and shortened my workout to the Basic Plus Workout for six months—and still kept losing inches! Now I'm a healthy size four—the smallest I have ever been. I'm eating more than I ever have, and I am much more active. My level of confidence has increased tremendously, and my self-esteem is the highest it has been in my entire life. Best of all, I am no longer imprisoned by diet and exercise!

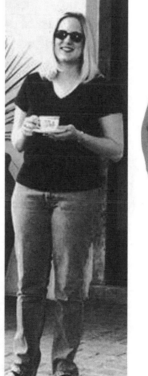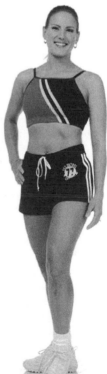

After being on the God-Made, Man-Made Food Plan myself for fifteen years, I have also tested it on thousands of T-Tappers, who have proven its effectiveness. Now it's your turn!

HOW THE GOD-MADE, MAN-MADE FOOD PLAN WORKS

- Spend two days consuming only God-made foods (see categories below). For example, enjoy meats, vegetables, soups, and salads, plus fruit in moderation. This is what I call "eating clean." It's always best to buy organic, but that can get expensive. Fresh is next best—just be sure to wash everything well before you consume it to get rid of pesticide residue. Frozen is okay too (so long as no sugar is added), but try not to eat canned goods since these typically have preservatives.

- Day three is what I call your "cheat" day. Of course, you shouldn't go overboard. It's always best to eat man-made foods (especially carbs) in moderation. But do relax and enjoy the foods you love, and don't worry about eating man-made carbs. If you want a brownie, have a brownie. If you want pasta, have pasta. I believe it's all psychological anyway. When you tell your body that you can't have a cookie, then you really want a cookie all day long and try to satisfy that craving with other things—and typically, in the end, eat the cookie anyway. But as soon as you tell your body you *can* have that cookie, you're going to ask yourself, "Do I really *want* it?" and the answer may very well be no. It sounds simple, but it is oh so true.

- Learn to listen to your body. What does it *really* want? Initially, you may find that you eat more cheat treats, but as T-Tapp helps your body rebuild its primary functions—especially elimination—and you allow your body a two-day break from processed foods, your body will balance itself out so you know without a doubt what it needs and wants, without diet and deprivation.

- Get back on track after your "cheat" day by resuming eating God-made foods for the following two days.

Note: If you are trying to lose more than two clothing sizes, you can adjust the God-Made, Man-Made Food Plan by eating God-made foods for three consecutive days and enjoying man-made foods every four days instead of every three. But never go longer than four consecutive days without man-made carbs, because intense cravings can occur, making you more likely to binge. After four weeks, move to God-made foods for two days and then a day of man-made foods. Once you reach your goal, you can have man-made carbs every other day without guilt, and your body will not store them as fat!

T-Tapp's God-Made, Man-Made Food Plan was created to help rebuild your body's ability to process man-made carbs again. The reason this plan works is because you're giving your body a mini-break from man-made, weight-gain food types, which allows it to process and eliminate the preservatives and excess glucose you consumed on your "cheat" day. This way, your body never becomes overloaded, which allows it the ability to rebuild your metabolic process.

YOUR GOD-MADE, MAN-MADE FOOD PLAN GUIDE

How do you tell the difference between God-made and man-made foods? My rule of thumb is that anything you can pick, gather, milk, hunt, or fish is God-made. Let's face it, potato chips don't grow on trees! Of course, there are a few exceptions, so keep reading.

Obviously, fresh, organic, and wild foods are going to be your safest choices, since many of today's supermarket foods are treated with pesticides and hormones or carry PCBs and mercury. But I don't want you to obsess over "eating clean." So long as you purchase the freshest foods you can find (and afford) and avoid any foods with artificial ingredients on God-made days, your body will improve its ability to assimilate, digest, and eliminate all foods—even man-made ones.

While I'm sure you don't need tips on what to eat on your "cheat" days, here are some guidelines for your God-made days. For easy reference, I've categorized these into food groups.

God-Made Carbohydrates

Fruits, most vegetables, and whole grains are carbohydrates that do *not* cause weight gain, primarily because they are nutritionally balanced and have no preservatives or additives. Their balance of vitamins, minerals, and fiber promote digestion, assimilation, and elimination.

It's important to consume a variety of vegetables, since different types provide different nutrients. Try to eat at least two colors of raw vegetables a day. Also include dark green leafy vegetables several times a week, since these are super-rich sources of vitamins and minerals. Keep in mind that you do need a little fat with your vegetables to assimilate the nutrients—try grated Parmesan or sharp cheddar cheese, almonds, olive oil, or butter.

Certain vegetables such as corn and white potatoes have been classified as high-glycemic-index, which means they have a higher tendency to be converted to glucose quickly and stored as fat. My opinion is that these foods contain necessary nutrients for a healthy body. Since I've been a borderline diabetic for over eight years, I realized that I can enjoy these foods in moderation as long as I combine them with other macronutrients—protein, fat, and fiber. Fiber acts like a sponge, helping to absorb fat and excess sugar. Fat and protein put a lid on the amount of insulin reaction your body is going to produce. And that, in turn, lowers the conversion of insulin to fat and enables you to use the sugar you ate as energy fuel. That's why I always order my baked potato with sour cream and put butter on my corn. (It makes them taste better, too!) It's also why I prefer almond M&Ms to plain ones. But if you're concerned about these foods, just consume them on man-made days—don't eliminate them.

When consuming whole grains and breads, focus on quality. Whole-grain breads without preservatives are your best bet, as are brown rice, wild rice, and spelt. Oatmeal (whole oats, not the instant stuff) is another excellent choice. In fact, recent research reveals that

GOOD MENU CHOICES
ON GOD-MADE DAYS

Breakfast

• Steak and eggs

• Hot oatmeal made from steel-cut oats (aka Irish oatmeal) with real butter and cinnamon

• All-natural, whole-grain, high-fiber cold cereal (look for brands such as Alpen, Arrowhead Spelt Flakes, and Ezekiel)

• Whole-grain buttered toast (from the bakery section of your supermarket instead of your grocery store shelf) with 100 percent fruit spread. Also check the refrigerated section of your supermarket for baked breads without preservatives, such as Ezekiel or Manna breads

• Fresh fruit dipped in raw nut butter, or assorted raw nuts (my favorite three are Brazil nuts, walnuts, and almonds)

Lunch/Dinner

• Fresh or frozen beef, chicken, turkey, or fish (trim all visible fat; remove skin from poultry; no breading; boil, grill, roast, or broil)

• Whole grains of your choice, such as brown or wild rice, spelt, barley, or buckwheat (no quick cook grains)

• Non-cured pork (roast or pork chops)—stay away from ham, bacon, or sausage

• Fresh or frozen vegetables

• Salad greens with your choice of God-made toppings, such as carrots, tomatoes, cucumbers, nuts/seeds, or sprouts, but no croutons or processed salad dressings—instead, use olive oil and flavored vinegars or lemon and assorted herbs

• Fresh or frozen legumes or beans

Snacks

• Seeds (sunflower, pumpkin)

• Soy nuts

• Fruit or raw vegetables with a raw nut butter dip

consumption of whole-grain cereals, such as oatmeal, assists the body with easier weight-loss management, not to mention helping the body to regulate blood sugar and cholesterol.

Fruit is nutritious, but be careful with it, as overconsumption can be converted to fat. I like to refer to fruit as "God's candy" because of its high sugar content. Of course, certain fruits are higher in sugar than others. Apples, cherries, pears, and grapefruit are low-glycemic-index, whereas grapes, bananas, kiwis, and raisins are high-glycemic-index. That makes some fruits smarter choices than others. But don't avoid high-glycemic-index fruits you love; just add raw nuts when you eat them to balance the sugar.

On God-made days, you should limit your fruit intake to no more than two servings. Fresh is always best because it's loaded with fiber and antioxidants. Frozen or canned is okay, too, if no sugar has been added. Eat dried fruit in moderation, however, since most contain sulfur (a preservative), and their sugars are concentrated. Also limit consumption of fruit juices, as many of these are mostly water and sweetened with high-fructose corn syrup and most lack fiber, which makes them easier to overconsume. Carb overload, including from juice, is what creates excess insulin and fat conversion. For better balance, make a habit of eating some protein (like raw nuts) along with fruit or fruit juices to keep insulin levels in check. And drink only 100 percent fruit juices (check labels).

Man-Made Carbohydrates

White breads, pastas, cookies, candy, cakes, bagels, most breakfast cereals, chips, and crackers are carbohydrates that tend to create weight gain, *even if they are fat-free,* not only because the body easily converts them to glucose, which in excess becomes stored as fat, but also because of their chemical additives (such as preservatives, artificial flavors, and artificial colors), which complicate the body's ability to digest, assimilate, and eliminate. Therefore, greater amounts of glucose become converted and stored as fat in fat cells. Once existing fat cells are full, the body creates more fat cells. And as I said before, when fat cells are created, they are either empty or full—they never go away!

Protein

Chicken is God-made, but chicken salad is man-made. Fish is God-made, but fish sticks are man-made. Steak, ground beef, and home-cooked roast beef are God-made, but meatloaf, salami, processed roast beef slices, and bologna are man-made. Pork chops are God-made, but bacon is man-made.

For best results, stick with lean meats, poultry, fish, and beans, as these are lowest in fat. Prepare meats in low-fat ways by trimming away all visible fat, removing skin from poultry, and broiling, grilling, roasting, or boiling these foods instead of frying them. Season foods as much as you like, but otherwise try to eat them as close to their natural state as possible—hold the gravy!—on God-made days. Finally, on God-made days, it's preferable to cook your own meals at home. That way, you know exactly how everything was prepared.

Please note that obviously, organic meats, poultry, and fish are ultimately the wisest choices on God-made days. But any fresh products are a lesser evil than those that have been heavily processed or otherwise altered with man-made ingredients.

Even though nuts and seeds are high in fat, their nutritional value is also very high, and the body needs quality fat to better digest, assimilate, and eliminate. Always try to choose raw nuts and seeds over roasted ones, since roasting destroys nutritional content.

Dairy Products

Most dairy products—milk, eggs, yogurt, cheese—may be eaten on God-made days. In fact, the latest research reveals that dairy products help the body lose weight easier. According to the *American Journal of Clinical Nutrition,* a recent review of studies on this subject concluded that over several years, those who had the highest intake of dairy weighed the least. Scientists believe the credit goes to calcium's ability to slow fat cells' production of the hormone cortisol, which has been linked to weight gain, particularly in the belly area.

When shopping, choose dairy products that are produced without antibiotics, synthetic hormones, or pesticides. Most organic dairy products meet this requirement. I believe you should avoid fat-free dairy

MAKING SMARTER CHOICES
ON MAN-MADE DAYS

Although you shouldn't feel restricted by food choices on man-made days, there are certain man-made foods that are closer to God-made foods than others.

- **Breads.** In addition to choosing whole-grain breads (versus breads with processed flour), it's a good idea to choose breads with few or no preservatives. Breads that contain sprouted grains are also healthier, and multiple grains are always a better choice than just one grain. My personal favorites are Ezekiel and Manna breads.

- **Pastas.** Best choices are pastas made without preservatives (look in the refrigerated section of your supermarket). Also, artichoke, spelt, or whole-grain pastas are better than those made with processed flour. I recommend Vita Spelt whole-grain pasta, especially for those who are sensitive to wheat.

- **Breakfast cereals.** Whole-grains are obviously a better choice than processed, sugary favorites. Granolas without too much sugar, shredded wheat, and cereals with many grains (even Whole Grain Total) are preferable as well. Peace Cereal, available at most grocery stores, offers several organic, whole-grain, low-fat granolas without preservatives or artificial additives. Vita Spelt offers a tasty whole-grain granola that is good for those who are sensitive to wheat, and Bear Naked offers a variety of very tasty, whole-grain granolas without preservatives or artificial additives that are soft, not crunchy, like most other granola cereals.

- **Cookies and cakes.** Grandma was right: homemade is best. When baked from scratch, these treats have fewer if any preservatives, additives, and artificial ingredients. And when eating packaged cakes and cookies, avoid those that contain trans fat.

What's so bad about trans fat? The vast majority of trans fats—also known as trans-fatty acids—are created artificially by bubbling hydrogen gas through vegetable oil, a process called partial hydrogenation. This transforms some of the oil's unsaturated fat into trans fat, which helps stabilize the oil (making it useful for deep frying and for packaged foods) and solidify it (making it suitable for margarine and many baked goods).

For years, researchers have referred to trans fat as the "stealth fat" because it lurks in a multitude of foods, and until January 2006, it wasn't required by the FDA to be listed on food labels. Numerous studies conducted by the National Academy of Sciences' Institute of Medicine have offered proof that trans fat not only increases blood levels of low density lipoprotein (LDL) or "bad" cholesterol, but—worse—actually lowers levels of high density lipoprotein (HDL) or "good" cholesterol. It has also been shown to cause major clogging of arteries, type 2 diabetes, and other serious health problems.

• **Candy.** Smarter choices contain the fewest ingredients. Hard candies or jelly beans, for instance, are better than nougats or candy bars. Plain dark chocolate or chocolate with nuts is better than milk chocolate or chocolate with creamy centers. In fact, those with diabetic or glycemic issues should always consume a raw nut simultaneously with candy, since combining the candy with a protein that contains fat will slow the absorption of sugar in your body and minimize its damaging effects.

• **Chips and crackers.** Baked chips are best, and again avoid trans fat. More and more food companies are offering these—not just for health reasons, but because they taste good. Personally, I think chips made with olive oil are delicious. Baked crackers that are trans-fat-free are a smart choice, as are whole-grain, rice, or seed crackers. I recommend Mary's Gone Crackers, not only because they are a quality, whole-grain, organic product with no hydrogenated oils or trans fats, but because they are also wheat-free and gluten-free.

products, however. These tend to contain more sugar, so reading labels is important. Most important, yogurt and sour cream needs to have live acidophilus and bifidus cultures, as these are good bacteria that help your body digest, assimilate, and eliminate.

Some guidelines: butter is God-made, but margarine is man-made. Cheddar cheese that has been naturally aged is God-made, but American slices or processed cheeses are man-made. All hard, naturally cured cheeses, such as Parmesan or Romano, as well as cheeses made from goat's and sheep's milk—like feta—are better choices than soft cow's milk cheeses, such as brie or cream cheese, on God-made days.

If you have a dairy allergy or are a vegetarian, products such as soy milk, soy cheese, and soy yogurt, as well as tofu, tempeh, miso, and so forth are good alternative choices.

Sugar and Fat

Consume foods high in sugar—even God-made honey and dried fruit—in moderation on both God-made *and* man-made days. And on God-made days, be sure to avoid any foods containing high-fructose corn syrup or artificial sugar.

When it comes to sugar, I believe it's all about choosing the lesser evil. For example, I recommend using turbinado or cane sugar and honey on God-made days and saving white or brown sugar for man-made days. Quick cheat treat: when you consume white or brown sugar, eat some cinnamon with it. Research shows this lessens your body's insulin reaction to sugar. Also, I would much rather see you eat real sugar than artificial sweeteners or laboratory-created sugars—such as high-fructose corn syrup—because your body can recognize it and process it.

In terms of fats, if you're trying to lose excess inches, it makes sense to consume these in moderation every day. But fats aren't necessarily bad. In fact, you need them for optimal metabolic function.

On God-made days, stick with high-quality fats such as extra-virgin olive oil, virgin coconut oil, and pure butter. Olive oil—another European staple—is a particularly good choice because numerous studies have shown that meals prepared with it can keep hunger at bay for up to five times longer than other meals. Recent animal studies also suggest that olive oil increases the activity of certain chemicals that "tell" the body to burn excess calories (through the release of heat), rather than store it.

I recommend drizzling olive oil on salads or using it to sauté or stir-fry vegetables. But keep in mind that cooking with olive oil at high heat—past its smoking point—not only destroys much of its nutrient value but can also cause it to become carcinogenic. Clarified butter (ghee) and virgin coconut oil are better choices for cooking at high temperatures. Since these have a higher smoking point and so don't break down as easily, they are noncarcinogenic—and I've found all of these to be very effective at controlling sugar cravings and helping with elimination.

On man-made days, you needn't be too concerned about restricting fats, with one exception. I strongly advise avoiding trans fat. Now that dietary guidelines require all foods to list trans fat on labels, it's easier to keep track of this previously hidden ingredient found in so many man-made foods.

Beverages

Drink your water! Water not only aids in hydration and weight loss, it also helps the body with better digestion, assimilation, and elimination. Tie your water intake to your body weight—take your body weight in pounds, halve that number, and aim to drink that number of ounces of water each day. For example, if you weigh 200 pounds, try to drink 100 ounces of water a day. Or if you weigh 120 pounds, try to drink 60 ounces of water each day.

Other beverages permitted on God-made days include unsweetened hot tea (herbal or regular) or coffee (with or without caffeine). But avoid drinking soda on God-made days, and *always* avoid drinking diet soda because of the artificial sweeteners. To me, a real soda is a lesser evil than a diet soda, so I often enjoy an occasional soda or two on man-made days.

- **Celebrate life!** Don't worry about consuming man-made carbs on your birthday, holidays, vacations, and other special occasions. In fact, you can consume those "forbidden carbs" every day for up to four days without disaster. Just return to the original two days God-made, one day man-made for a week or more. Then you can go back to every other day without worry.

- **Read labels!** Beware of processed energy bars, granola bars, and prepackaged diet meals. These are considered man-made because they all contain additives and preservatives.

- **Get fresh!** Fresh foods are always best for your body, so eat whatever is in season. These contain necessary digestive enzymes as well as optimal levels of vitamins and minerals. Try to make soups when vegetables are in season, then freeze these to enjoy in later months.

- **Get your fill of fiber.** As a rule of thumb, when foods get processed, they lose their fiber. Everyone knows how fiber helps the elimination system, ultimately giving you an internal workout so that food doesn't become stagnant in the digestive tract and leave you constipated. Fiber also absorbs toxins and waste products, then carries them out, so you don't store them in your body.

High-fiber foods—fruits, vegetables, nuts, and whole-grain breads and cereals—have not only been shown to prevent heart disease and many cancers, they also appear to fight obesity. One recent study found that young adults who ate at least 21 grams of fiber per day gained, on average, eight pounds less over a ten-year period than those who ate the least amount of fiber. Fiber definitely satisfies your appetite and keeps you feeling full for longer. Fiber has also been proven to help balance the body's reaction to simple sugars by using them as fuel instead of converting or storing them as fat.

The U.S. Department of Agriculture recommends we all get 25 to

30 grams of fiber per day. On days you can't get enough, I recommend taking a supplement to help the body help itself. And the best supplements? In my opinion, psyllium is an excellent soluble fiber, and it can be found in products like Metamucil, Fiberall, and Fibertox.

- **Savor every bite!** Whenever you sit down for a meal, try not to eat so fast that you barely taste your food. Slow down and enjoy every morsel. On man-made days, in particular, eating should give you a feeling of freedom. Remember, no guilt—enjoy!

The God-Made, Man-Made Food Plan gives your body its necessary components (protein, carbohydrates, and fats) to rebuild, repair, and eliminate. After you rebuild your body with T-Tapp and achieve your desired goal, you only need to do a T-Tapp workout two or three times a week and follow the God-Made, Man-Made Food Plan every other day to maintain your results.

Best of all, the combination of the T-Tapp workout and God-Made, Man-Made Food Plan allows you to eat without guilt and never diet or deprive yourself again. As I've said before, life is too short not to enjoy good food!

Frequently Asked Questions

7

Since launching T-Tapp twenty-five years ago, I have received thousands of letters and e-mails with specific questions about the workout. I've selected the most common inquiries to share with you.

Q: *Is the T-Tapp workout safe for kids?*
A: Absolutely. T-Tapp is safe for *all* ages and fitness levels, and as I always say, it's never too early or too late to get fit. As you probably know, obesity among children has recently reached epidemic levels. In fact, experts estimate that 15 percent of today's children are overweight, and another fifteen percent are at risk for becoming overweight. I believe T-Tapp can go a long way in helping to reverse this disturbing trend. Even thin children can benefit from T-Tapp because being thin does not equate to being fit.

Q: *Do I have to diet to get good results with T-Tapp?*

A: No, dieting is not required. In fact, I recommend that you not diet at all during the first few weeks of starting the workout. Instead, I advise consuming an additional 200 *high-quality* calories per day so that your body has an appropriate level of premium fuel at its disposal to rebuild muscles and body systems.

Q: *I love it that T-Tapp can be done at home on my own timetable, but where can I go if I need encouragement and support?*

A: Log on to my Web site (www.t-tapp.com), where you'll find forums filled with T-Tappers from all over the globe who are quick to offer advice and encouragement. Did you know that several studies have found that people who have support groups—even in cyberspace—lose three times as much as those who try to go it alone? Check my Web site often, as I often run sixty-day challenges. Prizes vary from a private workout session with me, a fly-in to a fitness retreat, or a makeover with a professional stylist, makeup artist, and photographer. But even more important than prizes, most T-Tappers enjoy these contests because it makes them accountable, increases their success rate, and motivates them to achieve their desired goals quickly.

REAL PEOPLE, REAL RESULTS

Kat Richter

"I started T-Tapping at seven years old."

My mom, Emily, is a T-Tapp trainer, and I started T-Tapping when I was seven years old. At first, I was weak in the knees because I had very long legs and a short torso. I even banged my chin with my knee doing Hoe Downs because my legs were so long. Now I am thirteen years old, and I have a lot more strength because of T-Tapp and swimming. My body type is now a Combo bordering on Short Torso.

Teresa Tapp has taught me so much about life and health. I thank her for making me how strong I am today.

Q: *Are there any T-Tapp classes or trainers in my area?*
A: Possibly. For a list of T-Tapp trainers, check the "T-Tapp Team" link at my Web site (www.t-tapp.com). My trainers and I also travel around the United States offering clinics and seminars. For a list of upcoming events, check the "Events" link at my website.

Q: *I have a bad back and problem knees. Can I still do the T-Tapp workout?*
A: Yes you can! In fact, T-Tapp's rehabilitative approach to fitness can help to rehab your problem areas. Remember, many of my signature moves were developed to help me deal with my *own* back pain! Even those who have had hip replacements can safely do T-Tapp, although I recommend starting with only two to four repetitions of each exercise, doing the workouts very slowly to focus on form, and working to the best of your ability. I have many testimonials from T-Tappers with knee or hip replacements who have not only improved their condition, but enjoyed inch loss as well.

Q: *I haven't worked out in years. Will I still be able to T-Tapp?*
A: Definitely. T-Tapp is all about working to your personal max. All that's required for success is to do your best with each and every workout. You start where you are, and as you gain strength and flexibility, you can add more moves and/or do more repetitions.

Q: *I've been lifting weights three times a week for about a year. Can I still do that and T-Tapp at the same time?*
A: As you begin to T-Tapp, I recommend that you focus on T-Tapp alone for three to four weeks. I've found that's the best way to achieve optimal results.

Q: *Does T-Tapp replace my other workouts, or can I T-Tapp in conjunction with them?*
A: T-Tapp is all you need to get (or stay) trim and feel terrific. So yes, it can replace your other workouts. However, if you enjoy other workout programs, you can apply T-Tapp principles (body alignment, KLT) to maximize their effectiveness.

Q: *I seem to have balance problems in that one side of my body feels stronger than the other—especially when I work out. Does this mean I should do more repetitions on the weaker side?*

A: No. T-Tapp moves will help correct these imbalances, but for optimal results, you need to do equal numbers of repetitions on each side. Otherwise, your problem could get worse.

Q: *Will T-Tapp help lower my cholesterol?*

A: I believe it will. Though I have no scientific evidence to prove this, I can tell you that many T-Tappers have received this health benefit. One thirty-eight-year-old client recently e-mailed me to report that her husband's cholesterol was well over 250 and that his doctor wanted to prescribe medication. Instead, she had him do my fifteen-minute Basic Plus Workout for two weeks—and guess what? His cholesterol dropped to the normal range!

Q: *Is it safe to T-Tapp in bare feet?*

A: Yes, but I don't recommend it—especially in the beginning, when you're developing better muscle density, strength, and flexibility at the knee, ankle, and base of the foot. Since I consider the feet to be the foundations of fitness, I advise supporting them in a good pair of cross-trainers. These will help provide support for your ankle and arch so that your body can maintain better alignment and you'll get better results.

Q: *I recently visited your Web site and was impressed with how many T-Tappers there are. How come I've never heard of your workout before?*

A: My focus has always been educational, not commercial. I've had many opportunities to do infomercials, but I've always declined. Instead, I chose to bring T-Tapp to the masses with a book. I believe a book gives me the ability to go into greater depth and provides consumers with a reference tool they can refer back to, so they can dig deeper and learn more.

Q: *Would you consider T-Tapp to be a "fusion" fitness workout?*

A: Definitely. T-Tapp incorporates elements of dance, yoga, Pilates, and more. But it's T-Tapp's stance and sequence of moves that elevate it to a class of its own.

Q: *This is an embarrassing question, but here goes. Does T-Tapp make you more regular?*
A: Yes! T-Tappers often say that T-Tapp and TP (toilet paper) go hand in hand. That's because when you work the body, layer by layer, with full fiber activation, plus pump the lymphatic system, intestinal organs are muscularly activated. As a result, these muscle contractions literally accelerate the elimination process.

Q: *Can I do T-Tapp while pregnant, and if so, for how long?*
A: You can T-Tapp through your *entire* pregnancy, but always check with your physician first. I have a Mommy Fitness section at my Web site, which offers trainer support from those who did T-Tapp while pregnant. Many have also achieved great results with postpregnancy shape-up by T-Tapping.

Q: *I'm seriously considering having gastric bypass surgery. Is it safe for me to do T-Tapp?*
A: I believe that T-Tapp will not only help your body better prepare for surgery, it can also help lessen the incidence of complications after surgery. T-Tapp can help accelerate your body's ability to heal, repair, and rejuvenate as well. Loose skin is the most common complaint following gastric bypass surgery, but T-Tapp can help you tighten and tone—plus you'll get that girdle effect.

Q: *I have more than a hundred pounds to lose. Can T-Tapp help me?*
A: Yes! T-Tapp was designed for all fitness levels, and I've had hundreds of success stories of T-Tappers who have lost more than a hundred pounds. But since your body's joints are carrying extra weight, I encourage you to focus on doing the best form you can as opposed to doing eight repetitions of each exercise—at least initially. Since I also understand the additional health issues that accompany those of size, I recently released a version of T-Tapp called T-Tapp MORE. It's a work-

out that's specifically designed for those who have more to lose and is available at www.t-tapp.com.

Q: *Since my teenage years, I've suffered from horrible PMS and muscle cramping each month—to the point of inactivity. Can I do T-Tapp?*

A: Not only can you, I'm convinced that once you begin T-Tapping, you should see an improvement in these areas within a month. You should also continue to see improved hormonal results as long as you continue to T-Tapp two to three times a week. The reasons for this are twofold: first, T-Tapp increases the body's ability to better balance glucose, insulin, and estrogen, and second, the girdle-tight muscles T-Tapp develops seem to improve the elimination of the uterine lining, which typically translates into less cramping.

Q: *Do I need to take any supplements while T-Tapping?*

A: A good multivitamin certainly can't hurt, but I also recommend taking alfalfa—not only because it's a plant protein that helps the body build muscle tissue, but also because it's clinically proven as an anti-inflammatory agent that will offset any newfound muscle soreness you may experience in the first two weeks of doing T-Tapp. For best results, alfalfa should be organic and pesticide-free. It should also be processed immediately after harvest to maintain the highest nutrient content.

8

Encore! Encore!

T-Tapp has so many success stories that I felt compelled to share more with you. My intention here is that as you read this book, you will find at least one success story you can relate to or identify with. Since all the success stories in this book focus on various stages of development and feature all body types, I hope you'll find several that inspire you, because as you begin T-Tapping yourself, I want you to realize that *yes you can,* too!

Ally Hoagland

"Mark my words, I will never again wear a size twenty-four!"

When I started T-Tapping, I wore a size twenty-four pants and had way too many rolls of flab covering my otherwise very sexy five-foot-eleven frame. I have the good fortune to be born with Dutch heritage (Teresa calls this one of the supermodel lineages) and a Combo body, meaning I have good bone structure and I gain weight evenly all over. No one ever believes me when I tell them how much I weigh because I look proportionate. However, anyone that has had the pleasure of wearing size twenty-four pants and having them get tight can tell you that proportionate or not, this is not fun. Shopping becomes so tedious, as you are left to decide between the dazzling dress with sequined swans or the brown and pink horizontal-striped turtleneck and accompanying stretch pants that don't stretch in the right places and for some maddening reason zip in the side or back.

I am only twenty-eight years old and I'm blessed to have no serious health problems. It was the shopping that motivated me to lose some sizes, but if I had let a few more years pass I would surely have ended up diabetic and with compromised health like my dad.

I lost a size in the first two weeks and I was only working out every other day along with some light walking on my in-between days. As soon as my twenty-twos fit comfortably, I took my size twenty-fours and did things to them—bad things. No way was I going to keep those hanging in my closet just in case I needed them again one day. Mark my words, I will never again wear a size twenty-four!

By the end of ninety days, I had lost two sizes and fifty-three inches overall! I did not spend hours a day working out. I did not adhere to some crazy diet. I tried to follow Teresa's God-Made, Man-Made Food Plan, until I reviewed my food journal and realized I had more man-made days than God-made days. Then I stopped worrying about that and simply tried to make better choices—like oatmeal for breakfast instead of a muffin, grilled or broiled fish instead of fried. I didn't count, measure, weigh, or exclude anything from my diet (except ice cream, because I'm addicted).

I also noticed improvement in areas that you simply can't measure by numbers. I am currently gearing up to start my last year of law school. I also work a full-time job. My stress levels are awfully high. Before T-Tapping, I was continually wondering why I felt so bad all the time. I'd never made the connection between working out and mentally feeling better. Now I know that T-Tapp is as much a workout for the mind as it is for the body.

My digestion and what happens after digestion are greatly improved as well, not to mention these lean muscles that keep showing up in cool places. When I T-Tapp regularly, my stress is manageable. I can handle all of my responsibilities so much more easily. A set of Hoe Downs in the middle of the afternoon or between classes or right when I am ready to doze off reading law books at midnight does the trick. It really is that simple. I also think I have developed what is known as the T-Tapp Glow. Someone actually told me that I looked radiant. Now that *is a compliment.*

I know the remaining sizes I want to lose will be gone just as quickly as these first few sizes. All I have to do is just keep T-Tapping! See photos in color insert.

REAL PEOPLE, REAL RESULTS

Emily Richter

From patient to success story to T-Tapp trainer!

For virtually my entire life, I have suffered from a variety of medical conditions. As a result of their impact on my life, it became a passion of mine to uncover the secrets to achieving optimum health. I strongly believe that if it were not for T-Tapp and my faith in God, I would have become permanently disabled and unable to help others who face their own battles.

At three years old, I was diagnosed with immune thrombocytopenic purpura (ITP) and hospitalized for three weeks. ITP is a disorder of the blood involving the immune system, and its cause is unknown. Antibodies, which are part of the body's immunologic defense against infection, attach to platelets in the blood (cells that help stop bleeding) and cause their destruction. ITP weakened my immune system from that point on.

At fourteen, I began suffering from chronic Epstein-Barr virus (CEBV)

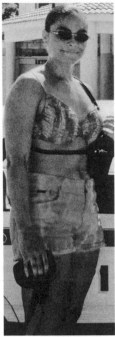

after an appendectomy and was bedridden my entire freshman year. After my fifteenth birthday, I began walking every night with my mother, which resulted in more energy, and I started eating more protein and whole foods. After six months of good nutrition and exercise, thankfully, the virus went into remission.

One month prior to my college graduation, at twenty-two years of age, I had to have a hysterectomy due to cervical cancer. Within three months after the surgery, due to hormonal imbalance, I had gained forty pounds and four dress sizes and was thrown into early menopause. For the next four years, I stayed in the gym six days a week, two hours a day, but with no success. Traditional exercise just wasn't enough to combat the cumulative effects of all my body had experienced.

In 1998, I discovered T-Tapp. This workout was able to do for me what four years in the gym could not. After only eight weeks, I had returned to my normal weight, shape, and energy level.

Since 2002, I have had three surgeries, one of which was a double mastectomy. After the surgery, I did as many T-Tapp movements as physically possible. Although it was a very emotional and painful surgery, my doctors could not believe the rate at which I healed. In addition to T-Tapping, within four months I was doing African dance and jazz dance and swimming laps—all of which require major upper body flexibility and strength.

In 2000, I decided to become a certified T-Tapp trainer. It is so rewarding to teach men, women, and children about nutrition and the T-Tapp system, and to help them overcome their own health and weight issues. I specialize in helping women who are going through or experiencing signs of menopause, as well as those who are struggling with obesity.

I am blessed that I am alive and on my way to greater wellness. I have a beautiful, healthy daughter who understands what it takes to overcome hardships and remain thankful. Yes, it has been hard, but all of it is worth it if I can be a blessing to someone who may be going through a similar situation.

Robert Mecham

"The joke was on me!"

After my wife showed me a few T-Tapp moves, I agreed to get up at 5 a.m. to support her new fitness goals. I remember thinking, "How challenging could this stuff really be?" and chalked up T-Tapping as the equivalent of sitting through a chick flick for the one you love. Wow, was I ever wrong. This workout kicked my butt! After sixty days, I'd lost 16.5 inches (5 inches off my waist). Not only did I feel better, but friends were commenting that I actually looked taller—probably because my posture had improved.

Guys, you owe it to yourself to give T-Tapp a try—just to see how in shape or outta shape you really are!

And gals: bet the man in your life that he can't T-Tapp. Chances are, after losing some weight, he'll come up with some new fitness goals of his own.

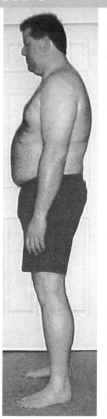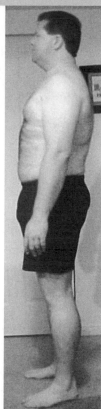

Sylvia Hoffman

"Everyone wanted to know what had happened to my 'Rice Krispies knees'!"

I began T-Tapping a couple of years ago after seeing a picture of the overweight, out-of-shape person I had become. I had seen the dramatic results this workout can bring on someone I knew, but I didn't think I would be able to do it because I had a very bad back (herniated discs) and bad knees. Besides, I hated to exercise!

My friend tried to convince me that the program was supposed to be reha-bilitative for back and knees, so I decided to try it out. I lost several dress sizes and many inches on that journey. Unfortunately, at that point, I was diagnosed with massive osteoporosis and was told by my physical therapists that it was so bad I shouldn't even be bending over to tie my shoes! I brought my tapes to the therapists and told them I really didn't want to give up this wonderful exercise program that had already made me feel so much better. Indeed, it had helped my back, my knees, and my energy levels, and I looked good for the first time in a long time. I knew after personally having these results that T-Tapp would have to be a part of my life.

Once I was given the okay to T-Tapp, things were progressing nicely when I forgot my limitations and started lifting 4 × 8 sheets of plywood. I fractured my lower back, and the pain sent all of the muscles in my right leg and my glutes into constant contraction. I had extreme nerve pain as well. Needless to say, I was unable to walk, sit, bend, or T-Tapp for a long time.

Once I started back, after two weeks of just doing Basic Plus, I was feeling better than I had in months. As I added in more exercises, my headaches and sinus problems disappeared. I felt more energetic, and I was also able to do more basic household chores. As I climbed the stairs of my house, I noticed that my knees felt better again, and there was no longer any cracking and snapping with each step that I took. Everyone wanted to know what happened to my "Rice Krispies knees'!" Overall, I lost eight inches in just two months. See photos in color insert.

Rose Riggs

"T-Tapp has brought me so many welcome life changes."

I heard about T-Tapp on my local PBS station. I caught just the last three min-utes, but that was enough to pique my interest. It looked simple. I'm not very co-ordinated, so complicated exercise videos just frustrated me. I was walking for exercise at the time, which made me feel good but did nothing for my stomach. I am the mother of five children, and my stomach was a blob.

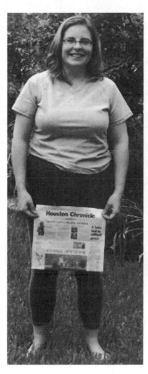
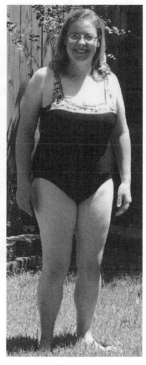

After a six-day boot camp, during which I really focused on my form, I noticed a huge difference. When Teresa said to hold my stomach in, I could do it—something I hadn't been able to do for five years!

Life has changed in many ways since I started T-Tapping. For years, I hated for people to even touch my shoulders because it hurt so badly. Now I am free to be hugged without pain. And I can let my toddler ride on my shoulders without shoulder pain, neck pain, or a headache. I can sneeze without crossing my legs—need I say more? I had been on and off antidepressants for years, having been diagnosed with severe depression, but since I began T-Tapping, my moods have been the most stable they have ever been with or without medication. This is such a relief, and I am so grateful—as is my husband. I lost my stomach "apron." The skin has tightened, stretch marks have faded, and even a scar from having my appendix out 25 years ago has disappeared!

Brenda Armendala and Theresa Broughton

Buddies build better bodies

THERESA: *My T-Tapp journey began with a bet between myself and Brenda Armendala. We were both fighting the battle of the bulge and felt determined that a little competition might just be the fuel we needed. Brenda kept telling me that she was going to reach her goal first, and I'd laugh and tell her that I would beat her no matter what. Actually, we both came out winners.*

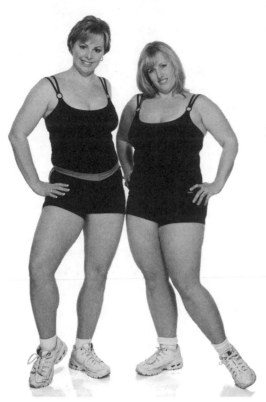

Prior to starting T-Tapp, I had a hysterectomy and major abdominal surgery for scar tissue. I was unable to do any kind of exercise for three months because of the surgery and recovery. Not only that, I had a scar with fat rolling over it like an apron. I wondered how I could possibly get rid of what I called my "whale meat." I felt certain that I would be spending hours at the gym. Thank you, Teresa Tapp! Within two months of T-Tapping, I had lost nearly eighteen inches and gained a passion to tell everyone I knew about how I'd done it.

This program helps with all of your muscles, working from the inside out. And for those who think that having a hysterectomy will affect their sex life, I have good news: tuck butt, knees out, KLT, and shoulders in alignment! I am so happy and so very thankful. I plan on T-Tapping for life.

BRENDA: *Before I started T-Tapping, I never thought I would ever feel my stomach muscles again. I honestly thought that I would be a big girl forever. I thought I should just accept it.*

T-Tapp was my last hope. Right away, I loved the workout, but I knew I would do better if I had a friend to keep me motivated. Theresa Broughton was very enthusiastic about T-Tapping, and we have inspired each other to continue working out. As a result, we have exceeded our expectations. I feel great. I actually like to get dressed in the morning, and my long-term goal is to wear a bathing suit without a bathing suit wrap!

Donna McWillie

There was an old gal about fifty,
Who was thinking she looked pretty nifty.
But "before" pics don't lie—and she started to cry—
'Cause her butt, well, it needed a "lifty."
But this Texan we'll call Donna Kaye,
Started Tapping the Lady T way.
She's engaging her lats, waving bye-bye to fat,
And the inches keep melting away!

See photos in color insert.

Terri Devillez

"In less than one week, I not only felt better, I noticed I had more energy!"

I have been battling my weight since junior high school, when I wore a size four-teen or sixteen. But I really started getting heavy after the birth of my son in 1981. Due to several factors, twenty years and two daughters later, I wound up wearing a tight size thirty-two.

My husband and I went to my company Christmas party in December 2001. I was really looking forward to going because I had bought a new outfit and really felt like I looked great. We had our pictures taken by a professional photographer at the party and I couldn't wait to receive them. When they arrived in January, I was mortified. All I could do was cry. I hadn't realized that I was really that big. I knew what my clothing size was, but before then it hadn't sunk in that my weight had gotten that much out of control.

I officially started T-Tapping in February 2002 with a fourteen-day boot camp, doing it to the best of my ability. Before the first week was up, I not only felt better, I noticed I had more energy. I had also lost nearly eight inches. By the end of the first month, I had lost over eighteen inches, and by the end of two months, I had lost over twenty-three inches.

The last time I measured (about a month ago), I had lost sixty inches and five pants sizes. I can now get on the floor and play with my two daughters and not worry about how I am going to get back up! See photos in color insert.

Sharlyn Bertrand

"T-Tapp gave me a new awakening about exercising and eating healthy."

I'm one of those who was always going to lose those extra pounds after January 1. Oh, did I say January 1? I meant by my birthday in June. Oh, June—well, that came too quickly this year. How about if I fit into that red dress again by next *Christmas? Is Christmas here already? I can't possibly diet with all this great food and parties. . . .*

This has been my cycle for at least twenty years. Lots of times I was able to lose a lot of weight, but I put it back on so quickly that I know my body didn't have time to recover.

T-Tapp finally gave me a new awakening about exercising and eating healthy. When I first started the program, I weighed 245 pounds and was wearing a tight size twenty-two. I am only five feet one inch tall, so I was really struggling with all of this excess weight. I was also having difficulty just climbing the stairs to my house.

I do not own a scale or monitor my weight. I did have a doctor's appointment in June of this year, however. Of course, they had to weigh me first. When the scale registered at 180, I was shocked—for two reasons. How could I weight 180 and be wearing a size fourteen? When I used to weigh 180, I was at least a size sixteen. Oh yeah . . . T-Tapp! Okay, I will take the size fourteen (almost a twelve now) and the 180 (or whatever it is by now). My goal was to be in a size ten, but now I'm thinking that since I'm so short, my new goal should be a size eight. Although I have lost weight before, once I got to a size fourteen, for some reason, I would quit and balloon back up to the plus sizes again. I have been at a size fourteen for a couple of months now, so for me, knowing that I am going to continue on to a goal is a whole new wonderful life-changing experience.

See photos in color insert.

Connie Tindall

"I finally got my lifetime wish: a flat stomach!"

I have always struggled with keeping my tummy flat, but entering menopause really thickened my midsection—especially when I went on hormone replacement therapy. I felt like I had lost control of my body. Even the books I read concerning menopause informed me that it was only natural to gain weight and that I should just accept it as part of the aging process.

What complicated my situation further was that I had a prolapsed uterus, and my doctor wanted to perform surgery. For eight months, I went to a local gym, often doing a combination of weight training, lunge classes, and aerobics up to four to six hours a day—all in an effort to prevent surgery and lose weight.

I started to lose some weight, but felt like my stomach was not budging—even after doing a hundred sit-ups a day! I also felt consumed with working out at the gym and had little time for anything else. Even my daughter, son, and husband began to complain. When I found T-Tapp, I finally began to understand the mechanics of my body. I am a Short Torso and learned that I don't have much room for my internal organs. As my body type ages, those internal organs drop south and expand outward due to weak internal muscles. We need muscles to act as girdles—to hold those organs in and to achieve maximum results for a flat stomach, those organs need to be put in place prior to muscle movement.

With T-Tapp, I also learned that by doing so many sit-ups a day, I was creating a hard, round tummy. But it wasn't until I started putting my organs in place that my abdomen shrank over an inch in just one week!

I recently returned to my physician, only to discover that I no longer needed surgery! Furthermore, my hormonal mood swings have balanced out and I no longer have dramatic food cravings. After five months of T-Tapping, I've also gone from a size sixteen to a size eight and lost over twenty inches.

See photos in color insert.

Paul Collier

"I now have the energy to keep up with the teens I help at my church."

I've always been a big guy, so when I started T-Tapp, I wasn't expecting miracles. Besides, I was more focused on getting my health and blood pressure under control—especially since my mom had just died from complications from her chronic high blood pressure. In two weeks, I felt better and started to look better. In four weeks, the cellulite on my arms and belly were gone! In two months, my blood pressure was normal, and I had to buy new clothes. Best of all, I now have the energy to keep up with the teens I help at my church. I can do "Dance, Dance Revolution" as good as—if not better than—any of them! See photos in color insert.

Laura Huerta

"Just when I thought I'd be disabled for life . . ."

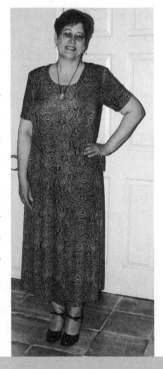

My T-Tapp journey actually began over four years ago when I first read about this program in Woman's World *magazine. At the time, I was recovering from a car accident in which I had suffered whiplash and a back injury. Although initially attracted to the program because I needed to lose weight (I had not been able to work for three months after the accident), I searched for T-Tapp's Web site to learn more about its benefits. I was very pleased to learn that there were exercises specifically aimed at helping with back conditions.*

I dove right in! Within a week, I knew I'd hit on an exercise program that would change my life. T-Tapp Twist ended up being the exercise that helped my spine recover from the accident. Within three weeks' time, my back felt nearly like new—just when I thought I'd be disabled for life! An added bonus was that I lost twenty-five pounds and countless inches (I don't know exactly how many, because I'd started the program for health reasons and didn't measure) within five months and felt better than I had in a long, long time.

Nearly a year later, my health began to deteriorate, and I gained back the twenty-five pounds and inches I'd lost. Eventually, I was diagnosed with gluten intolerance. My reading on this condition helped me to understand that my small intestine could not absorb vitamins, minerals, or hormones properly. For that reason, I had developed severe iron anemia, vitamin deficiencies, and hormonal imbalances throughout my body. I also learned that it would take between six and twelve months for my body to recover and be able to absorb everything properly again.

Little by little, as my health began to improve, I began to add T-Tapp back into my life. Once again, T-Tapp came through for me when my health was poor and brought me back from what I refer to as a "disabled" state of mind. At both times in my life, I felt as though my situation was hopeless and that doctors could no longer help me. Although I consider myself a work in progress, I know that if I continue to T-Tapp, take my gluten-free liquid vitamins and iron, and allow my body to return to a state of balanced hormones, my health will continue to improve. That body, by the way, is now thirteen pounds lighter and has lost over thirteen inches in the past two months. T-Tapp has handed me back my life!

Shannon Keefe

"I'm far shapelier now than I was a decade ago!"

As a teenager I broke my hip, and I've had some minor problems associated with that injury in the twenty years since. I also have scoliosis, and as a child I had physical therapy for it. I had been noticing this year that the ribs on my left side

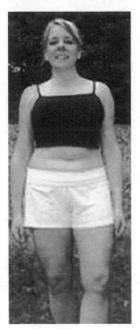

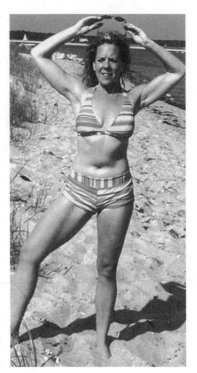

were starting to protrude as if my back was twisted. This worried me a lot, but I tried to keep my mind off it. As I got more serious about T-Tapp, I eventually noticed that while my left side is still not quite even with my right side, it's much more in line with it now.

I have had minor problems with my weight since just after high school, and for me, it was truly lack of exercise and bad eating habits. At age twenty-two, I wore a size five and weighed 122 pounds. Now, at thirty-four, I weigh 132 pounds and wear a size six or an eight. But I'm far shapelier now than I was a decade ago! See photos in color insert.

REAL PEOPLE, REAL RESULTS

Janice Metcalf

"I found new muscles and a new awareness of linear alignment that made me feel wonderful!"

"Thunder thighs" was the affectionate name I was called growing up. From an early age, I rarely had a positive self-image, and I always compared my physical attributes to those of other girls, which left me feeling inadequate. These comparisons sidelined me, as I became a people watcher instead of an active participant in normal high school activities like sports. I have always felt chunky.

Well, "chunky" continued through young adulthood, and my body even started to add extra weight, despite all my efforts to exercise regularly and eat

low-fat foods. Marriage and two beautiful daughters later, I continued to strug-
gle with my size and weight. A dark cloud also hung over my head with a fam-
ily history of heart disease, high cholesterol, high blood pressure, and diabetes. I
believed these conditions were my destiny as I struggled with being the "average"
size twelve or fourteen, which was too big for my frame.

Desperately searching answers, I stumbled onto the T-Tapp Web site quite
by accident. I started to read everything there and thought Teresa was sending
me a private message, "Yes you can," so I started on my T-Tapp journey. Right
away, I found new muscles and a new awareness of linear alignment that made
me feel wonderful. My self-confidence improved, and I felt stronger. I have never
enjoyed exercising so much. Then the inches began melting away. My records
show a loss of twenty-one inches, and I was wearing a size eight in about nine
months.

Over time, however, I stopped paying attention to form and indulged in
way too many man-made foods, and the inches crept back on. Wearing a size
twelve again, losing the motivation to move and always feeling lethargic, I went
to my doctor for an annual exam. Casually mentioning my "always tired" phe-
nomenon, he requested that I have my thyroid checked. To my surprise, I was di-
agnosed hypothyroid with Hashimoto's disease.

Over the next eight weeks, I tried to work out in the morning and then
again in the afternoon for about fifteen to twenty minutes at a time. Then I
started doing just morning workouts sporadically, but usually did Primary Back
Stretch and Hoe Downs every day.

Within eight weeks, I was down six and a half inches and eating a little
bit healthier every day. I now have a new outlook on life and truly believe in
Teresa every time she says, "Yes you can" and "You did it!" because I am *doing*
it. In fact, I am feeling great and showing my daughters the T-Tapp way.

See photos in color insert.

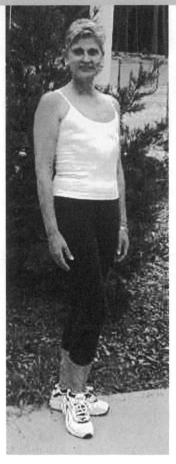

Sybil Janke

This breast cancer survivor T-Tapped her way through treatments

After T-Tapping for about six months, I took a life-changing detour with breast cancer. Following my double mastectomy/lymph node surgery, and during the chemotherapy and radiation treatments, I continued to T-Tapp as often as possible. I credit this exercise program with helping me to regain complete flexibility in my arm and keeping my compromised lymph system working well. In addition, while others might have started to lose correct posture after such a surgery, mine has remained erect and aligned.

T-Tapp not only does all of the cosmetic things it is advertised to do, it has been a great benefit to me in my recovery from cancer. I am almost five years out from cancer surgery and continue to attend T-Tapp classes. Fifty-three and still cancer-free. Thanks, Teresa!

Grace Remer Spriggs

"T-Tapp helped me fit into my wedding dress!"

I love T-Tapp because it has changed my way of thinking about my body. I have never had a weight problem, but I have long had a problem with my body image. Being one of the tallest girls in my grade and having (undiagnosed) scoliosis, I developed bad posture early in life. Even though I was naturally slender, when

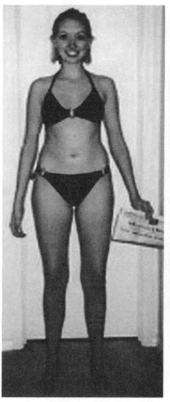

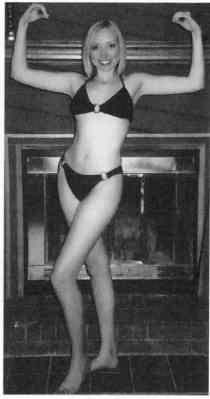

I looked at myself in the mirror, I saw myself as fat. I did all kinds of exercises I found in magazines. Not only did my body not change, but my back hurt so bad that I couldn't even finish most of them. So for years—from age fifteen to twenty-one—I hated the way my body looked and began to believe that was the way it was going to have to be.

Then I began to T-Tapp regularly. Almost right away I noticed little changes in my body—like my stomach slimming down and my back and shoulders becoming toned. I started reading on Teresa's Web site about different body types and what they were capable of achieving. During the workouts I could feel myself getting stronger and accomplishing moves I had not been able to do before. Slowly, my brain opened up to the idea that my body is unique and that I am an individual. I realized that I could not change my height or the length of my legs and arms. I also realized that I had a choice. I could spend even more years obsessing and dreaming of another body, or I could embrace what God had given me and recognize how beautiful I truly am. T-Tapp also helped me realize that I need to respect my body and have realistic expectations when I work at enhancing the good things and not try to morph myself into something I can never be.

Oh, and one more added bonus: T-Tapp helped me fit into my wedding dress better and have a body I was proud to show off for my new husband without feeling insecure.

Jeni Huffstedtler

"My baby fat disappeared with T-Tapp!"

While pregnant with my daughter, Lillian Hazel, I tried to do a full length T-Tapp workout twice a week beginning at week fifteen. The only move I omitted—at thirty-two weeks—was Lawn Mowers, because the bending to the side and down seemed to make the baby uncomfortable. I also tried to do four sets of Hoe Downs per day to help with circulation and lessen my chances of water retention. T-Tapping during pregnancy was hard sometimes, but I felt much stronger and more alert when I did it.

My labor lasted only three hours and fifty minutes! I used some T-Tapp techniques during labor to help me cope. Arching my back during contractions and holding my abs tight and tucking my tush during the peak of the contractions helped a lot!

I began doing a mini-T-Tapp workout six days after giving birth. I did Organs in Place, Half Frogs, Primary Back Stretch, Oil Wells, T-Tapp Twist, the Lunge Sequence, and Hoe Downs for a while. I have lost thirty-seven inches and over thirty pounds since Lily was born. My arms and legs are in better shape than before pregnancy. It's hard to find time to work out with a young baby around, but I try to do a full workout three times per week. And it's definitely paying off! See photos in color insert.

Sue Fetzner

"I have truly been blessed, and my whole life has changed."

I was diagnosed with fibromyalgia in 1990, after many years of suffering without a diagnosis. I had also been in two car accidents that aggravated many of the symptoms I was already dealing with. For over fifteen years, my life was haunted with pain from head to toe: migraines, digestive problems, sleep distur-

bances, sleepless nights, chronic fatigue, extreme lack of energy, infections, candida, lack of muscle control, muscle spasms, feelings of hopelessness and worthlessness, mental fogginess, and challenges with weight gain. I would flinch from pain when someone touched me. Most mornings I had difficulty getting out of bed due to the pain and stiffness, and many times I crawled on the floor as I started my day. My own and my children's daily activities were adversely affected on a regular basis. I tried to hide my pain and problems from others. My family didn't understand what I was going through and many times everyone thought I was "making it up." It was very frustrating because you look okay, but you don't feel okay. This elevated the anxiety and stress, which made everything worse. I found it difficult and sometimes impossible to be much of a person, a mom, or a wife.

By August 2000, my condition had worsened and reached a point where I was occasionally using crutches, had limited use of my hands, was taking $2,000 worth of meds a month, was unable to work, and had difficulty taking care of my family and household or participating in any activities outside my home. Two specialists told me that I would soon live my life from a wheelchair. I was on the road to permanent disability and living a life with excruciating pain. At one time I had been a teacher but now could not pursue this career, or any career for that matter, because I could no longer get through a workday. I also lost my own small business partly due to my health challenges. By this point my husband and I faced constant financial problems due to the expense of my treatments, medication, and inability to work. Taking many pharmaceuticals and seeking constant medical attention and therapies was part of my daily routine. Over and over again I was told that there was nothing that I could do and that my body would continue to deteriorate. My life was falling apart before my eyes, and I was running out of hope.

Then someone told me about T-Tapp, and my life has not been the same since. When I first started doing the workout, I could only do it for a few minutes. Gradually, my body became stronger and healthier, and I started to drop sizes. I didn't expect that to ever happen because I'd been told that I was too old to ever get a young-looking body back and that I just had to accept the fact that I was aging. But with the results that I was experiencing with T-Tapp, I knew that I was on to something. My body was rebuilding, reshaping, and getting stronger, and I was feeling great.

I now live an active life—free of discomfort—and am able to maintain a high level of fitness and body conditioning without much time and effort. No one ever guesses my age. I am forty-nine years old, look much younger, and feel like I am twenty again. I am a mother of three, and I have returned to a size four from a ten or twelve. T-Tapp is a part of my daily routine. I do some of the exercises every day. I do not diet, but do mostly follow Teresa's God-Made, Man-Made way of eating. I am mentally sharper, more energetic, physically stronger, and more focused in my purpose than I have ever been. I no longer take pharmaceuticals and haven't made a visit to a doctor for any health challenges for almost five years. I am active all day, work full time with my own business, and enjoy traveling and being active with outdoor activities such as swimming, hiking, skiing, boating—whatever I want to do. I have truly been blessed and my whole life has changed. See photos in color insert.

Molly Chambers

The healing powers of T-Tapp

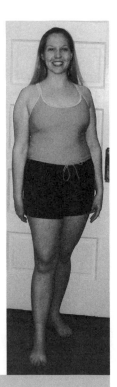

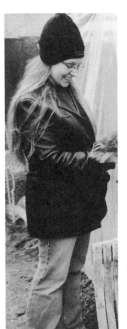

The T-Tapp workout originally appealed to me because of its rehabilitative approach. I was desperate to find an exercise program that would allow me to rehabilitate a knee injury. I had been to five different physical therapists, and not one concurred with any of the others in terms of the appropriate therapy. The only thing they all seemed to agree on was that I couldn't exercise like I wanted to.

I was given the choice of surgery but wasn't keen on the idea, since my doctors assured me that surgery would entail developing arthritis in the next ten or twenty years. Meanwhile, my knee pain continued. In fact, one leg began to swell while the other atrophied—not a pretty sight! One leg was almost an inch bigger than the other!

Worse yet, the pounds were creeping up as I struggled to find an exercise program that I could do without worsening my injury. I had almost given up on the idea when I found T-Tapp.

This workout has left me pain-free! It has also helped to even out my legs! I'm getting trimmer, too—most noticeably in the lower abdomen (yeah!). I can actually feel muscle in my arms and tummy instead of fat. My schedule thus far has been to alternate between the Basic Plus Workout and the Total Workout each day, taking one day off each week. Some days I've wanted to work out more, but I've noticed that I have a tendency to overtrain or even add inches when I work out too much. So it has taken a little discipline to work out this little and still see results!

Jane Heinrichs

"I feel like a new woman—inside and out!"

When I started T-Tapping in February 2003, I had a multitude of health problems stemming from a broken tailbone at age seventeen. Constant leg, back, and neck pain—along with total adrenal failure—had really compromised my quality of life to near nothing. But I was so happy when I

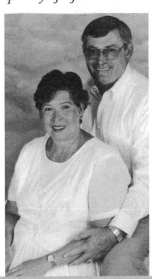

managed to complete the fifteen-minute Basic Plus Workout— even if I did have to take three days off between workouts (due to exhaustion from my adrenals). By Thanksgiving, I had so much to be thankful for: 80 percent of my spinal and joint problems and discomfort had improved, and I had little or no pain in my neck. Even friends and family noticed how much

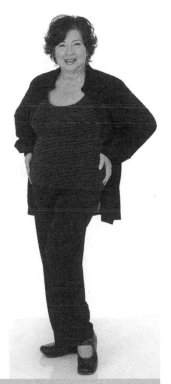

better I could move, and I was still just managing to do the Basic Plus Workout two or three times a week.

By October 2004, I was able to do Basic Plus, as well as a few additional moves from the Total Workout, several times a week. These days, I'm working out as much as five days a week and have my energy and vitality back. I credit T-Tapp and rhodiola (a daily supplement my doctors prescribed for my adrenals) for this amazing turnaround. I feel like a new woman—inside and out—and the fact that I've dropped three clothing sizes in the process is just icing on the cake!

REAL PEOPLE, REAL RESULTS

Scott Broughton

"I couldn't believe it—my belt needed a new hole!"

What can I say? I didn't even measure when I started T-Tapp. I was only trying to help my wife by working out with her in the morning three times a week. I didn't diet and my weight didn't change, but when I put on my suit for my son's banquet, my belt needed a new hole! In eight weeks I lost four inches from my waist. At fifty-one, most men have a hard time losing from their waist, but I'm a believer now! See photos in color insert.

REAL PEOPLE, REAL RESULTS

Dr. Rosario Martinez-Castillo

T-Tapp provides a psychological boost

I am a psychotherapist and work for a community college in the Houston, Texas, area. Working in the college atmosphere and being married to the president of a university means that I have to entertain quite often, as well as attend functions, so it is important that I always look my best.

I used to buy each of my outfits in three different sizes so that no one would know if I was up a size or down a size. With T-Tapp, I am now in my smallest size and no longer have to worry about gaining it back. But part of what helps me feel better is knowing that exercising speeds up my metabolism and gives me a sense of well-being. The last thing I want to do is exercise after a busy day, but making myself do that enables me to feel reenergized and able to go out in the evening and have a guiltless dinner. It is just a psychological boost.

Of course, it also helps when your husband is a T-Tapper, too. Mine rehabilitated his shoulder by T-Tapping and now uses the workout to stay fit. See photos in color insert.

Lani Muelrath

"People tell me that I look younger today than I did five years ago!"

As a T-Tapp trainer with five years of practice, I continue to be astonished by the results I get for so little investment of my time. This is exactly what I wanted for myself and my students: a powerful, smart exercise approach that would deliver health and beauty all at once with minimal investment of time and maximum investment of intelligence in movement.

I came to T-Tapp with over twenty-five years of experience as a fitness teacher and trainer. I was at a point in life where I wanted to get the most out of my time investment in exercise and not have to work out all that much to get it! As a very busy working woman, this is a priority.

About three years prior to T-Tapp, I had become certified in and was specializing in Pilates. This was the most effective technique that I had found to date. Then I came across T-Tapp, which I recognized had a synergism that topped everything else I had done.

The changes, personally? The most dramatic effect on posture I have experienced from any other practice. Reshaping of my already fit physique: trimmer torso, more graceful lines through my arms and legs, lifting in key places, joint stability and comfort, and tremendously maintained flexibility and aerobic endurance. Is it any wonder I choose to specialize in T-Tapp? It continues to be a deep pleasure to bring the same gifts of health and beauty that I have received from this practice to an ever-expanding circle of students! And people tell me that I look younger today than I did five years ago! See photos in color insert.

Deborah Baker

From doom and gloom to sheer success!

Before I started T-Tapping, I was on several medicines (maxed out on oral diabetes medicines and about to be put on insulin, plus taking Tenormin for irregular heartbeat and Lipitor for high cholesterol) and could barely bend over to tie my shoes.

Then I began to focus on eating in a healthy manner and incorporating daily exercise into an almost completely sedentary lifestyle. In just five months, I was completely off all medicines and had drastic improvement in my mobility.

In 2003, I had two surgeries for breast cancer—one in May and another in June. The following year, I had knee surgery and soon after that broke my foot in three places. As a result, my transformation has been a slow process and I'm definitely not there. Still, knowing how desperate I felt before, I hope to be an encouragement to others who find themselves in similar situations. Never give up!

See photos in color insert.

Dorothy Trahan

T-Tapping at 80 and looking good!

I discovered T-Tapp in Prevention *magazine in April 2003. I tried the Hoe Downs that were featured in that article and found them quite challenging.*

I have exercised regularly since age eighteen, when I was diagnosed with scoliosis. I was told by an osteopath that if I didn't do something, I would be a hunchback by the time I was forty. Although that seemed to be eons away, I followed his directions, which were to put a bar in the bathroom door and hang on it every time I went to the bathroom.

In my fifties, I started doing Callanetics. After a while I found them boring, and because I was in good shape for my age, and life got in the way, I was not doing much of anything.

Then one summer, I went to buy a new bathing suit and definitely did not like the image that stared back at me. My waist was big, my butt was gone, and I had a stomach that would not suck in. Where were my hip bones? Looking at pictures taken on vacation, I saw that my shoulders were slumped and my head stuck forward. Where was the person that I had always known and been pretty proud of? This was a picture of an elderly woman. I was getting old, but not gracefully.

Then I discovered T-Tapp. I have had wonderful success with this workout in a very short time, and my body seems so happy to be working again!

I think all seniors should T-Tapp. I believe it will not only enrich their lives but perhaps prolong it. By the way, I had my eightieth birthday last January, and didn't get home till 3:45 a.m.! See photos in color insert.

Ginger Breinig

"I've lost five sizes without being a fanatic!"

I am a five-foot, eight-inch redhead with a secret. Although I weigh 195 pounds, I'm only a size twelve! How is that possible? I attribute it to a little thing called muscle density.

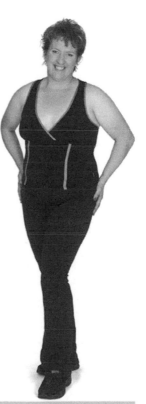

Thanks to T-Tapp, I weigh thirty pounds more now than when I was this same size ten years ago—before having my kids. Pretty amazing, isn't it?

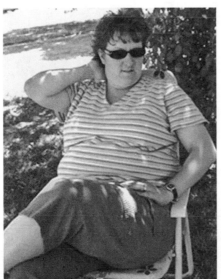

I've been T-Tapping off and on for three years or so, and for the most part, too much off and not enough on! I tried and tried and tried to do the fourteen-day boot camp, assuming that's what I had to do to be a "real"

T-Tapper. Well, anytime I did a boot camp longer than four days I would get physically exhausted, emotionally overwrought, and just plain yucky. Then, upon "failing" to complete my boot camp, I'd be depressed and upset, and then not T-Tapp for three weeks. Hmmmm, didn't get me anywhere, did it?

When a dear friend and fellow T-Tapper pointed out to me that I only needed to do four days of boot camp, I remember thinking, "Yeah, right, like that's going to be enough to help me lose at least four sizes." But she was right! The more important aspect of T-Tapping is consistency, or the every-other-day routine that comes after boot camp. Proof this works? Well, in one year, I've lost five sizes!

Do I exercise every day for hours at a time? Hardly! I have a very busy life. I do aim for two to three forty-five-minute T-Tapp workouts a week, with shorter fifteen-minute workouts added in on most alternate days. But I always take off at least one full day a week.

I do my best to add T-Tapp principles to other areas of my life as well—like engaging my lats when I drive. Not all the time, mind you, but I try for five miles on, followed by a couple off. And I tuck my butt, too, of course. I figured out that I could load and unload the dishwasher while in KLT position, and that makes cleaning the kitchen even more of a workout than it already is!

T-Tapp has truly changed my life. I look at my body differently now, I look at clothing differently now, and I live my life better now. I'm also a better wife, mother, and friend because of it.

Appendix

Available at T-Tapp.com

T-Tapp Basic Plus Workout* (45 minute instructional, 15 minute workout). This VHS or DVD set contains two workouts—one with detailed instructions and one without instructions, along with the "Yes You Can" seminar (90 minutes) that teaches you how to use T-Tapp techniques in daily activity.

T-Tapp Total Workout* (15 minute Basic Plus and 50 minute Total Workout). This VHS or DVD set contains three workouts—one with instructions (48 minutes) and two without instructions, along with the "Yes You Can" seminar (90 minutes) that teaches you how to use T-Tapp techniques in daily activity.

T-Tapp Tempo (27–55 minutes) (Regular, Intermediate, Arms, Torso, and Lower Body). Designed for the experienced T-Tapper, these VHS or DVD workouts contain new movements and sequences of movements to specifically target areas of concern and yet still be a full body workout. (T-Tapp Tempo workouts are only available to customers who can show proof of purchase of *Fit and Fabulous in 15 Minutes* or those who have purchased the T-Tapp Total Workout.)

T-Tapp MORE Workout (40 minutes and 20 minutes). This VHS or DVD contains two workouts, with and without instructions, and is designed for those who have more to lose, more health problems to overcome, and/or more birthday

*The T-Tapp Basic Plus and Total Workout are featured in this book.

candles on the cake. The tempo is slower, the exercises are modified from the original Basic Plus and Total Workouts, and there are fewer repetitions. T-Tapp MORE is designed to rebuild cardiac health, neurokinetic pathways, and lymphatic function, as well as deliver body sculpting, inch loss, and weight loss.

T-Tapp MORE Rehab Program (80 minutes). This VHS or DVD set contains four 20-minute workouts, with and without instructions, plus rehabilitative instructions for daily activity (how to go up stairs without knee pain, etc.). Originally designed for people of size, this program is excellent for those with health issues (frozen shoulders, bad backs, knee problems, and arthritic conditions), as well as for those who have more birthday candles on the cake (degenerative spine and joint issues usually increase with time without proper movement). Take the first step in rebuilding your health, wellness, and fitness with the T-Tapp MORE Rehab Program—you'll get MORE results in less time!

Step Away the Inches Walking Workout (22 minutes). This VHS or DVD aerobic walking workout provides cardiac conditioning and total body sculpting—especially arms—without any jumping, kicks, or equipment. Discover the difference in walking the T-Tapp way and learn how to maximize inch loss with any walking program.

Step It to the Max (50 minutes). This VHS or DVD walking workout contains more upper body movements and step/lift sequencing for increased core cardio concentration. In addition to form tips, it also contains T-Tapp warm-up and cool-down stretches for comprehensive conditioning.

Hit the Floor (30 minutes). This VHS or DVD workout uses T-Tapp sequencing along with gravity to develop abdominal muscle density with the power to pull organs in and up. It contains all new exercises, like Organs in Place/Half Frogs, not featured in Basic Plus or Total Workout. The T-Tapp Hit the Floor workout is one of the most comprehensive abdominal workouts on the market today, and even very fit clients are amazed at how challenging this workout is.

Hit the Floor Softer. This VHS or DVD abdominal workout was created to use with or without weighted shoes. The original Hit the Floor exercises have been modified to allow the body to progressively develop muscle density and strength without strain or compromise of form. Form tips taught at end of workout help maximize effectiveness—even when applied to regular version of Hit the Floor.

Hit the Floor Combo. This VHS or DVD set combines both Hit the Floor and Hit the Floor Softer into one package for significant savings.

Hit the Floor Harder (52 minutes). This VHS or DVD workout is more comprehensive and definitely more challenging. It begins with exercises from the first ten minutes of Total Workout and finishes with form tips after the workout to optimize inch loss from waist to knee. (This workout is only available with proof of purchase of T-Tapp Total Workout or *Fit and Fabulous in 15 Minutes.*)

T-Tapp Mundial. T-Tapp Workouts are available in Spanish in VHS or DVD, along with e-mail and telephone (*en español*) support as well.

T-Tapp Deaf/Hard of Hearing. T-Tapp workouts for deaf/hard of hearing are translated in American Sign Language and are closed-captioned. They also come with e-mail and telephone support.

T-Tapp International. The T-Tapp Workouts are currently available in French, German, and Russian. Additional languages soon to come!

CRT Skin Tightening System. T-Tapp exercises work the muscles, but skin needs exercise, too! The CRT Skin Tightening System contains a body-brushing pattern designed to help the body help itself tighten, tone, and control cellulite. This package also includes a natural plant fiber body brush, a one-month supply of supplements to naturally nourish the skin (Premium Blend Alfalfa) and assist elimination of toxins (Fibertox), as well as bonus lymphatic exercises to help the body "battle the bumps." A complimentary copy of "The Truth about Cellulite" seminar also explains how cellulite control is possible without lotions, pills, or expensive treatments. The combination of CRT with T-Tapp enables the body to lose inches quickly without loose skin!

CRT Brochure and Body Brush. Just the basics for a better body. Depending upon age and amount of inches lost, supplements are not necessary for the skin to tighten and tone.

Premium Blend Alfalfa. Botanical nutrient supplement that can help rid the body of retained water and inflammation, as well as help the body function to correct problems associated with skin elasticity, cellulite, and hormonal balance. Premium processing elevates this source of alfalfa to supreme nutritional density.

Fibertox. Proprietary herbal supplement that can help stimulate the body as a machine to use its own elimination systems to help rid the body of toxins released from external stimulation.

Pyruvyl-Glycine Spray. This proprietary formula enables you to maximize your workout with endurance and fat loss by boosting your body's Krebs cycle. All ingredients are natural and nontoxic and do not increase heart rate or blood pressure.

References

Chapter 2: Yes You Can!

American Council on Exercise makes fitness trend predictions for 2005. http://www.acefitness.org/media_display.cfm?NewsID=208.

Anderson R.A., C.L. Broadhurst, M.M. Polansky, W.F. Schmidt, A. Khan, V.P. Flanagan, N.W. Schoene, and D.J. Graves. Isolation and characterization of polyphenol type-A polymers from cinnamon with insulin-like biological activity. *Journal of Agricultural and Food Chemistry*. 2004; Jan 14; 52(1):65–70.

Boosting your energy. http://www.health.harvard.edu/special_health_reports/ Boosting_Your_Energy.htm.

Campbell, W., M. Krim, V. Young, and W. Evans. Increased energy requirements and changes in body composition with resistance training in older adults. *American Journal of Clinical Nutrition*. 1994; 60:167–175.

Drexel, H., G. Lorvenser, P. Langer, T. Marte, C. Wielander, and C.H. Saely. Effect of concentric muscle training on glucose tolerance in healthy sedentary individuals. Abstract P35380. European Society of Cardiology, ESC Congress. August 28–Septmbcr 1, 2004, Munich, Germany.

Growing stronger: Research and background about strength training. http://nutrition.tufts.edu/research/growingstronger/why_grow_ stronger/research_and_background.html.

Guo, H.R., S. Tanaka, W.E. Halperin, et al. Back pain and prevalence in U.S. industry and estimates of lost workdays. *American Journal of Public Health*. 1999; 89: 1029–1035.

Luo, X., et al. Estimatcs and patterns of direct health care expenditures among individuals with back pain in the United States. *Spine.* 2004; 29(1): 79–86.

Overweight prevalence. http://www.cdc.gov/nchs/fastats/overwt.htm.

Stewart, W.F., J.A. Ricci, E. Chee, D. Morganstein, and R. Lipton. Lost productive time and cost due to common pain conditions in the U.S. workforce. *Journal of the American Medical Association.* November 12, 2003; 290(18): 2443–2454.

Chapter 3: Getting Ready to T-Tapp

Boschmann, M., J. Steiniger, V. Hille, J. Tank, F. Adams, A.M. Sharma, S. Klaus, F. Luft, and J. Jordan. Water-induced thermogenesis. *Journal of Clinical Endocrinology and Metabolism.* December 2003; Vol. 88: 6015–6019.

Grout, P. *Jump Start Your Metabolism: How to Lose Weight by Changing the Way You Breathe.* Fireside Press. 1996.

Lewis, D. *Free Your Breath, Free Your Life: How Conscious Breathing Can Relieve Stress, Increase Vitality and Help You Live More Fully.* Shambhala Publications. 2004.

Woodland, K.K., J.E. Benson, M.J. Luetkemeier, R.C. Bullough, R.G. Barton, and E.W. Askew. Dehydration: Does it influence resting rate? *Medical Science Sports Exercise.* 1996; 28:S43.

Chapter 6: The God-Made, Man-Made Food Plan

Consumers Union. The stealth fat. *Consumer Reports.* March 2003, pp 28–31

Gittleman, A.L., and B. Sears. *The Fat Flush Plan.* McGraw-Hill. 2002.

Hoffman, R.L. *Tired All the Time: How to Regain Your Lost Energy.* Pocket Books. 1996.

Jacqmain, M., et al. Calcium intake, body composition, and lipoprotein-lipid concentrations in adults. *American Journal of Clinical Nutrition.* 2003; 77:1448–1452.

Kroenke, C.H., N.F. Chu, N. Rifai, D. Spiegelman, S.E. Hankinson, J.E. Mason, and E.B. Rimm. Moderate alcohol consumption has beneficial glycemic effects. *Diabetes Care.* 2003. July; 26:1971–1978.

Ludwig, D.S., M.A. Pereira, C.H. Kroenke, J.E. Hilner, L. Van Horn, M.L. Slattery, and D.R. Jacobs. Dietary fiber, weight gain, and cardiovascular disease risk factors in young adults. *Journal of the American Medical Association.* 1999; 282:1539–1546.

Mediterranean diet found to be more effective than strict low-fat option. Press release. Friday, October 5, 2001. http://www.nuthealth.org/nutrition/med_diet.pdf.